Praise for *Mama: Love, Motherhood and Revolution*

"A SEMINAL PIECE THAT DRAWS A LINE IN THE SAND ON WHAT MOTHERHOOD SHOULD BE ALL ABOUT. It is a statement that has the potential to realign motherhood, and is so intelligently written. [It is] to motherhood what Germaine Greer was to womanhood."
– Dr. John Irvine, founder of the Read Clinic, best-selling author and child psychologist

"Motherhood is not only the root for the survival of our species, but also lies at the core of all human functions – biological, social, cultural, spiritual, economic, educational, artistic and every other aspect of human existence. In the context of our post-modern society, *Mama: Love, Motherhood and Revolution* is UNDENIABLY THE MOST IMPORTANT BOOK OF THE 21st CENTURY. It explores, with exquisite beauty, a magical and mysterious world of motherly being, fascinating and filial aspects of femininity, the developmental impact of being Daddy – for him and his child. The dysfunctions of our world emanate from the disastrous consequences of devaluing mothers and motherhood, sacrificed for sexual satisfaction, material benefits, and corporate profits in a male-dominated world. And thus, ritual replaces faith, tweets/text messages displace conversation, skimming or surfing the web substitutes for a depth of understanding, and a ceaseless chatter supplants the comfort of a loving silence. Humanity decides, often in retrospect, that 'civilization' or 'progress' were not all that they were made out to be, perhaps a return to our innate nature and natural ways may serve society better. Now is one such moment in time. *Mama* sounds the clarion call to return motherhood to its former glory, preserved for millennia but recently wrecked by the senseless onslaught of materialism, modernism and media.

"I could not have predicted the profound impact of *Mama*. While making rounds in the Paediatric ICU after reading it, I insisted that the entire team go into the patient's room, so that the mother did not hav
Later in the morning, I becam
nurse interposed herself betwe

obstructing the mother's attempts to calm her baby down during the removal of a breathing tube. Clinicians like me have consistently disarticulated the mother–infant dyad, dismembered the family dynamic that is crucial to healing and health, and imposed inviolate rules and policies to justify this insanity. No more of this, at least in my practice, will be tolerated."

– K. J. S. Anand, MBBS, D.Phil., FAAP, FCCM, FRCPCH, Nils Rosén von Rosénstein Laureate 2009, Professor of Pediatrics, Anesthesiology, Anatomy and Neurobiology

"ANTONELLA RAISES TWO REALLY IMPORTANT IDEAS. Firstly that we need to become an attachment society, so that the role of mothers especially becomes an easier one. And that we need to depolarize the thinking about attachment parenting, so that everyone can find themselves free to move on that continuum."

– Steve Biddulph, Professor of Psychology and #1 bestselling author of *Raising Boys*

"Love is the essence of life, the essence of flourishing and connecting, the essence of human growth and flowering. MAMA IS A LYRICAL ODE TO THE NEED TO LOVE AND A GUIDEBOOK ON HOW TO EMBRACE LOVE. This deeply inspiring and informing book about the empathic connection between mother and child reminds us of how much we need to nurture both mothers and children in their crucial roles of advancing humankind."

– Peter R. Breggin MD, psychiatrist and Director, Center for the Study of Empathic Therapy, and bestselling author of *Toxic Psychiatry* and *Psychiatric Drug Withdrawal*

"Part memoir, part social deconstruction, *Mama* at once embraces and wrestles with the phenomenon of modern motherhood, every second chapter or so seeing Gambotto-Burke rumbling with one of ten renegade experts who form a disturbing chorus. To suggest a patriarchal plot is not to be a fringe conspiracy theorist. In his 2012 book *Sex and Punishment*, Eric Berkowitz argued convincingly that ancient lawmakers, spooked by what they saw as the possibility of blokes becoming biologically redundant, had created a society that would condemn motherhood to little more than a masculine factory in which women laboured. This society exists today, motherhood still regarded as a temporary vocation for which one must seek 'leave', presumably from something more important than the raising of emotionally nourished human beings. Together, the voices in *Mama* push this same barrow, and it makes for an arresting argument. The author herself brings the mystery of motherhood up close and personal. Having lost a brother to suicide and her mother to a 'corrosive relationship', Gambotto-Burke watched her own daughter marvel at her first dawn and found it 'the most exquisite moment of my life' ... this is the experience of motherhood: PERSONAL, MAGICAL, SUBLIMELY POWERFUL, and medical jargon can take a hike. Gambotto-Burke's point is that the shared experiences of mothers are of a value no PhD can match."

– Jack Marx, *The Weekend Australian*

"What would a celebrated writer known for tackling themes as dark and intriguing as suicide, addiction, sexuality and celebrity culture make of something as supposedly tame and ordinary as motherhood? Antonella Gambotto-Burke's latest book, *Mama: Love, Motherhood and Revolution*, is part advice for new parents, part a call to arms for change and part memoir. In essence, though, it's about intimacy. A BOOK LIKE NO OTHER, it prepares the reader for an entirely new encounter with intimacy, that with their baby. It recognises not just our vulnerability around intimacy but also the ways in which intimacy calls upon our unresolved pasts. *Mama* is a celebration of attachment and our drive to overcome obstacles in the pursuit of closeness with our child, and shows why parental intimacy is neither tame nor ordinary."

– Andie Fox, *Daily Life*

"AMAZING, AMAZING ... Buy this wonderful book!"

– James Mathison, Channel 10

ALSO BY ANTONELLA GAMBOTTO-BURKE

Mouth

The Eclipse: A Memoir of Suicide

The Pure Weight of the Heart

An Instinct for the Kill

Lunch of Blood

Subscribe to Antonella Gambotto-Burke's blog at
antonellagambottoburke.com

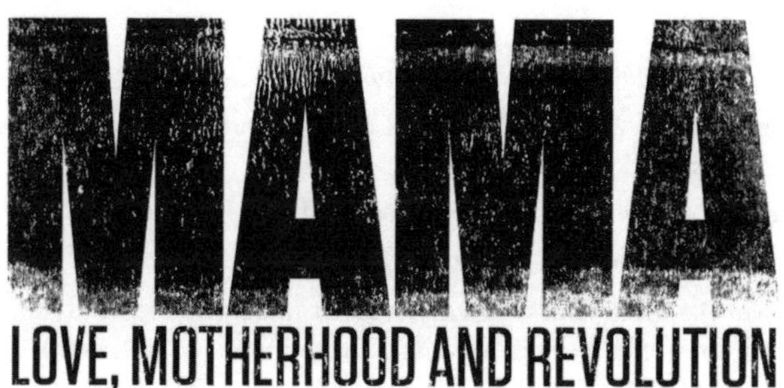

MAMA

LOVE, MOTHERHOOD AND REVOLUTION

ANTONELLA GAMBOTTO-BURKE

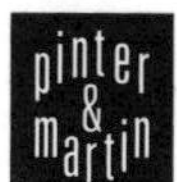

pinter & martin

Mama: Love, Motherhood and Revolution

First published in 2014 in Australia as *Mama: Dispatches from the Frontline of Love* by Arbon Publishing Pty Ltd.

This revised edition published by Pinter & Martin Ltd 2015

ISBN 978-1-78066-205-3

British Library Cataloguing-in-Publication Data
A catalogue record for this book is available from the British Library.

Set in Minion

Printed and bound in the UK Ashford Colour Press Ltd, Gosport, Hampshire

This book has been printed on paper that is sourced and harvested from sustainable forests and is FSC accredited.

Pinter & Martin Ltd
6 Effra Parade
London SW2 1PS
pinterandmartin.com

For Bethesda, forever suspended in
the space between my heartbeats:
this book was named for your first word.

So who mothers the mothers
who tend the hallways of mothers,
the spill of mothers, the smell of mothers,
who mend the eyes of mothers,
the lies of mothers scared
to turn on lights in basements
filled with mothers called by mothers in the dark,
the kin of mothers, the gin of mothers,
mothers out on bail,
who mothers the hail-mary mothers
asleep in their stockings
while the crows sing heigh ho carrion crow,
fol de riddle, lol de riddle,
carry on, carry on –

Chorus by Catherine Barnett

ANTONELLA GAMBOTTO-BURKE'S GUIDE TO MOTHERHOOD

1. Cherish your child. You could drop dead tomorrow. Chase them around the house and kiss them. Cuddle them. Write them cards. Draw them pictures. Tell them they make you happy.
2. Unplug the antenna. Use your television set only for DVDs and when your baby/toddler is asleep. Never, ever listen to the radio or loud music when your baby/toddler is around. Watch less TV, curb Facebook and stop tweeting. Why? Because nobody really cares.
3. Take your child for walks. Without your mobile. Without your iPod. And talk to them. Tell them about flowers and bugs and trees and clouds and sky and sea and your childhood. Be present. Connect.
4. Always always always hold your child's hand, even if it means wearing Birkenstocks. I wore Birkenstocks for six years. And maxiskirts. Walk slowly. Forget the rest of the world.
5. Be as fat as you need to be when your child is young. Do not listen to anyone who makes you feel bad about your weight. You can lose it when they're at school; I did. Eat cake.
6. Dance with your partner. In the kitchen. In the hallway. Especially in front of your child. The very best kind of dancing is when there's no music playing. Cut loose. Be free.
7. Avoid stressful people. This includes family and old friends. You have my permission. And if tempted to feel guilt, remember the impact of maternal stress on children: very, very bad.
8. Lie with your child in the dark after reading them a story. Talk about their day. Really listen. Don't stop reading and listening and talking in the dark just because they can read. Then push the blinds aside and look out at the stars together in the dark. And as you do, think of all the mothers who have lost their children and how fantastically lucky you are.
9. Start baking. There is no wound that a cake doesn't go some way toward salving. Banana, coconut and rum cake with cream cheese icing is the answer to just about everything. Truly.
10. Make friends with mothers in your neighbourhood. Find one that fits. Some are deeply peculiar but then you'll meet one who makes you laugh as she drives you to your first colonoscopy.
11. Buy or make bunting, and invest in sparklers. Love is a privilege, so celebrate!

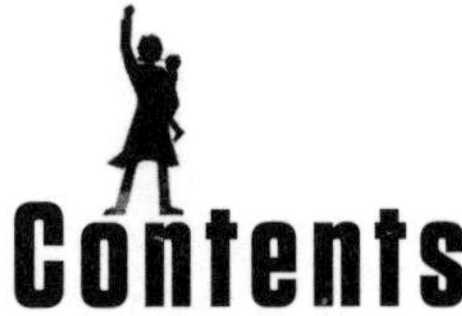

Contents

The language of love

Introduction by Michel Odent

The passion Antonella feels for her daughter is the golden thread that runs through every one of these pieces.

A French newspaper recently mentioned a project for reconsidering the vocabulary related to the national school system. The author of the article was analysing the reasons why the term "*école maternelle*" (school for children aged two to six) should be replaced by the term "*école première*". The vocabulary that has been used for nearly a century is suddenly deemed sexist, since it suggests that a young human being needs first his/her mother. On the same day, I read about the recent announcement of US Defense Secretary Leon Panetta that lifts the prohibition of women and mothers serving in combat. From now on, women and mothers are given the permission to kill, like men.

It is in this context that I began to read *Mama: Love, Motherhood and Revolution*, Antonella Gambotto-Burke's anthology of essays and interviews about femininity and motherhood. Through her transgenerational perspective, Antonella has found the most eloquent and concise way to be critical of our unisex society: we have, as she writes, reached a phase when "the denigration of femininity [is] everywhere". A gifted writer, Antonella needs only a few lines to turn our attention toward the essential. "Our culture", she writes, "is now one of masculine triumphalism, in which transhistorically feminine expressions – empathy, sweetness, volubility, warmth – are seen as impediments to a woman's professional trajectory".

Antonella brings an unusual slant to the subject: an

essayist, critic and journalist, she is also an attachment parent. Having decided to sleep separately, she then co-slept with her daughter until her daughter turned four. Warned that hers was the experience of birth associated by specialists with impaired attachment and postnatal depression, Antonella writes, "The possibility no professional volunteered was that through parenthood, my husband and I would experience the kind of romance that, for years, endured as bliss". After the birth, Antonella was wheeled, holding her newborn daughter, "past trees laden with baubles – it was the night after Christmas – and into a new universe that defied every law". Fascinated by this new universe, she interviewed me, Gabor Maté, Sheila Kitzinger, Laura Markham and others. She wanted to understand what motherhood means.

The passion Antonella feels for her daughter is the golden thread that runs through every one of these pieces, a love sourced in her own feeling for her "compassionate, emotional, gentle" grandmother, a woman whose talents, from the perspective of Antonella's peers, were "wasted".

And I can echo Antonella's words because I belong to the generation of her grandmother.

I have learned, from my own transgenerational perspective, that our cultural conditioning related to the men–women relationship can fluctuate at a high speed, like fashions. Let us illustrate from an example the speed of such fluctuations. Women who gave birth (at home, of course) around 1920 or 1930 used to say, "I cannot imagine my husband watching me when I was giving birth". They were thinking in terms of sexual attraction afterward. Some decades later, their granddaughters were saying, "I cannot imagine giving birth without my husband/partner".

Today, the basis of our cultural conditioning is that women can do all that men can do, and vice versa. Focusing on the differences and on the complementarities of men and women is "sexist" (pejorative). Scientific perspectives are becoming the best allies of common sense to neutralize the fast fluctuations of cultural conditioning. This is what I am learning from seminars and workshops for health professionals involved in childbirth.

The reactions of participants when I describe a situation

usually associated with an easy birth are telling: what happens, I ask, when there is nobody around a labouring woman apart from one experienced and silent midwife, perceived as a mother figure, sitting in the corner of a small, warm, dimly lit room, and knitting? This apparently simple scenario is unknown and culturally unacceptable in the context of the twenty–first century. I have the authority to describe its effects because I spent six months as an "externe" in the maternity unit of a Paris hospital in the early 1950s, before the advent of theories that are the bases of modern schools of "natural childbirth". A common reaction of participants is that promoting knitting is "sexist": knitting is supposed to be female. Other common questions are, "What about the father?" or, "What if the midwife is a man?" All these reactions are expressions of that which Antonella calls the "denigration of femininity". In general, my attitude is not to argue or to answer directly the questions; rather, I interpret this situation in the light of the latest physiological discoveries.

There are physiologists who are studying the effects of repetitive tasks such as knitting. We learn from them that knitting is a way to reduce the levels of adrenaline. Why is the level of adrenaline of the midwife important? An emerging discipline – the exploration of the "mirror neuron system" – is using sophisticated methods to demonstrate how contagious emotional states are, including emotional states associated with high levels of adrenaline. In other words, the knitting midwife is helping the labouring woman to maintain her own level of adrenaline as low as possible. This is essential since it is well known that the release of hormones of the adrenaline family inhibits the release of oxytocin, the key hormone during the birth process. All factors that can influence the level of adrenaline must be taken into account. The temperature of the room is one of these factors. When the midwife has good experience and is perceived as a mother figure, it is probable that the mother-to-be will feel secure – the prerequisite to avoiding an increased level of adrenaline.

Human beings are special where childbirth is concerned, because they have developed to an extreme degree the part of the brain called the neocortex – the brain of the intellect. An involuntary process such as the birth process can be inhibited by the activity of the thinking brain. This is why a labouring woman needs to be protected against stimulation of her neocortex. I referred to the silent midwife: language is the main stimulant of the neocortex. When we feel observed we have a tendency to observe ourselves: the neocortex is stimulated. This is why I mentioned a scenario with one midwife: it is much easier to have a feeling of privacy when there is only one person around. In many traditional societies they had proverbs claiming that when there are two midwives the birth is difficult. For the same reasons, we visualized the midwife sitting in a corner of the small, dimly lit room, rather than staying in front of the labouring woman and looking at her.

Such physiological interpretations of the effects of a situation offered as an example – not as a model – can easily lead the participants to comment on a paradox. Today, it is politically correct to be critical of doctors who prescribe too many drugs and perform too many caesarean sections. At the same time, situations that might make a birth easier are not culturally acceptable.

There are many ways to illustrate the current collusion between science and common sense. When I was a medical student in a Paris hospital around 1953, I had never heard of a mother who would have said, immediately after giving birth, "Can I keep my baby with me?" The cultural conditioning was too strong. All mothers were convinced that a newborn baby urgently needs "care": the baby was immediately given to a nurse. While staying in the maternity unit, babies were in a nursery. Mothers were elsewhere. Nobody had thought that they might be in the same room.

It is in such a context that we suddenly learned from scientific perspectives that a newborn baby needs its mother. What an important discovery! Some scientists introduced the concept of critical period for mother–baby attachment. Others looked at the behavioural effects of hormones that fluctuate during the period surrounding birth. Others looked at the contents of the colostrum. Others found that a human baby is able to find the breast during the hour following birth. Others studied childbirth from a bacteriological perspective and came to the conclusion that, ideally, the newborn baby's body should be immediately colonized by microbes transmitted by the mother.

Interestingly, even during the twenty-first century, there are still women who don't need the justification of sophisticated scientific perspectives to rediscover common sense. This is the case with Antonella, the mother of Bethesda, the little prodigy who could say "mama" at the age of four months. An opportunity to keep in mind that the Latin word "mamma" ("teat") has inspired the classification of Homo sapiens among "mammals", species characterized by the complementary roles of females and males. Babies can also help us to reintroduce common sense.

"I look at her, my heart everywhere", Antonella writes of her daughter. "Inviolate softness, made holy by capacity for feeling. This, then, is femininity, I think … Just this: a little girl, her mother, and the wind rippling through poplars."

Common sense is only one of the many reasons Antonella's writing about parenting has been published around the world. The depth of the devotion she feels for her daughter reminds us of what it is to be human mammals.

Michel Odent
London, England
wombecology.com

Motherhood in the twenty-first century

Foreword by Antonella Gambotto-Burke

Throughout history, the most brutal cultures have always been distinguished by maternal-infant separation.

Like almost every other woman I know, I once perceived motherhood as the consolation prize for women who didn't have what it took to make it in the workplace. In her mid-thirties, a girlfriend – now, ironically, a family-cultivating politician – dismissed mothers as "drudges" and "breeders". To us, being a mother was acceptable only if motherhood was not one's *raison d'etre.* As a sidebar mention, it passed muster; as a passion, it indicated only a paucity of capacity and imagination.

In the West, this perceptual template is now near-universal. The nurturance of a child is considered a squandering of the educated and the elite. Female high-achievers now hunger for "challenges" in place of connections. British economist Alison Wolf reported that women now make up the majority of undergraduates in the West. "There are now four women graduating with bachelors degrees in the US for every three men," she wrote. "In the UK, almost 60 per cent of students, at undergraduate and postgraduate levels, are female." An American study of Harvard and Radcliffe graduates demonstrated that women "increasingly delayed marriage as the decades progressed, and nearly 40 per cent of women in all three groups never had children at all."

The British Chancellor of the Exchequer recently referred to mothers raising their own children as a "lifestyle decision", as if it were on a par with nudism or polyamory. This perspective is reinforced by the behaviour of women we admire. A week after giving birth to her third son, Cate Blanchett – the most celebrated actor of her generation – was addressing a summit. Rachida Dati, a minister in former French president Nicolas Sarkozy's cabinet, returned to parliament *in heels* five days after a caesarean, a procedure now classed as major surgery. And actor Halle Berry, pregnant with her second child, said, "After giving birth I will go back to work as soon as possible. When I got Nahla I took time off for almost four years. But now that job-wise everything is going so well, I definitely want to keep on working." (Her depiction of babies as impediments to a woman's primary purpose is made clear by a related headline: *Halle won't let baby stop her*.)

Singer Lily Allen was similarly frank about her desperation to return to the unthreatening world of praise and objects. Of her two daughters, then under three, she said: "I love my children, but I'm a very impatient, busy person naturally so two babies, neither of them can talk, it was quite boring! … I missed the positive feedback about my music from my fans. I missed the rush of performing. I missed the free clothes and handbags and the good tables in posh restaurants. I did!'

Such responses are unsurprising given the menial status of motherhood. Our cultural take on both success and heroism – the ideals of any civilization – reflect a prejudice that is staggering in its latitude. Throughout human history, heroic conduct in particular has almost exclusively been attributed to men; women are generally only considered heroic in the context of wartime and even then, in token numbers. Despite the fact that heroism pivots on courage, self-sacrifice and the preservation of other lives, the billions of mothers who died in childbed have been forgotten.

Despite the mortal risk, there is no gravity attributed to motherhood. Instead, it continues to be almost universally disparaged by feminists and sentimentalized by men. In 2013, *four times* as many women died giving birth around the world than there were casualties in the Syrian Civil War, and yet there were no headlines, crisis bulletins, aid packages or expressions of public outrage. The 293,000 women who die in pregnancy and childbirth every year (and the seven to ten million who suffer severe or chronic illnesses caused by pregnancy-related complications) do so without public recognition of any kind. There is no statuary. There are no wreaths, medals, processions.

Presidents do not stand in silence for the mothers who have fallen.

It would be considered demeaning to present a veteran of war with bows and candy to commemorate his service, but women who have almost haemorrhaged to death, whose sexual organs have been irreparably damaged through episiotomies, whose bladders are perforated during c-sections, who have been rendered incontinent, paralyzed by epidurals, suffered Post Traumatic Stress Disorder after botched c-sections or spiralled into an incapacitating postpartum depression in the service of their families are presented with similarly infantilising tributes by their partners every Mothers' Day. (For those who consider such situations exceptional or outlandish: the US Agency for Healthcare Research and Quality reported that 94 per cent of American women who gave birth in 2008 had "some sort of pregnancy complication" resulting in an expenditure of US$17.4 billion).

The seriousness of childbirth on every level – emotional, spiritual, physical – for mothers is not only ignored, but effectively derided. "Congrats! You've had the baby … now what?" *Fitness* magazine trumpeted, before suggesting that "the general rule of thumb is to head back to the gym six weeks after birth". Implicit in advice like this – and it is everywhere – is the understanding that having a baby is an event like any other ("now what?"), that a mother's instinct to place her infant's needs before her own is old hat ("the general rule of thumb"), and that it is not only acceptable but correct for a mother to separate from her baby. The extent of this disconnection is made clear by the popularity of 000-sized onesies printed with the words, "Get off Facebook and feed me!"

Maternal–child attachment is mostly eroded in increments. The separation begins in hospitals, where mothers are not only made to feel inferior to medical professionals in relation to their infants, but regularly separated from their infants for examinations, bathing and so on. One mother I know remains traumatized by her experience of giving birth in an elegant private hospital. "My son's Apgar scores were actually very good," she said, "but he was immediately whisked off to NICU without me even having had a chance to greet him. They did wheel him past me on the way out so that they could tick the box that I had seen my son. While being stitched up, I thought: 'I feel like I have had my appendix out, not a baby.' I didn't get to experience my baby at all."

She was told that she wouldn't be able to see her premature baby again until the next day as they had no-one to wheel her to NICU. Despite having had a c-section, she was determined to spend time with her newborn son and, against all advice, staggered three floors down. "I just sat there talking to him and trying to touch him," she remembered. "I was forbidden from holding him. They repeatedly told me that I wasn't permitted to hold him because he was too fragile and it it was too much trouble to move all the equipment. And, as my son had no suck reflex, I was made to feel redundant by the staff. I was a nuisance; I got in the way of them performing their jobs. Bonding, love and warmth had no value to them at all." She wept as she recalled watching as a nurse almost ripped a strip of skin from her son's face as she removed the tape for his breathing tube.

Shamefully, human beings are the only mammals to separate mothers from their infants. Dr John Krystal, Professor of Psychiatry and Neurobiology at the Yale School of Medicine, described the impact of maternal separation on the infant as "profound", citing the recent discovery that the autonomic activity (heart rate and other involuntary nervous system activity) of two-day-old sleeping babies is 176 per cent higher during maternal separation. "We knew that this was stressful but the current study suggests that this is a major physiologic stressor for the infant," he concluded. The association of maternal–infant separation with developmental havoc is not new. Scientists have, for many decades, separated newborn animals from their mothers to study the resulting damage to the evolving brain. And yet despite the evidence, little difference has been made to the way mothers and babies are treated, both by hospitals and by society at large.

This separation has a trickle-down effect, resulting in a

disastrous chronological apartheid. Children are placed in care and then in school (in Britain, policy wonk Paul Kirby has gone so far as to suggest extending the school day from nine until six); adults work themselves into cardiac arrests alongside their coevals, and the old are stored in aged-care facilities until their expiry dates are up. That which is lost in the wash is love. There is a world of difference between the experience of "care" – the wiping of a bottom, the bathing of a body: basic biological obligations – and the intimacy that makes us want to live. Willingly, we are scripting simple happiness out of our lives.

Arguably the most destructive facet of this attitude is our cultural repudiation of maternal sensitivity, a quality that can only evolve through quiet, calm, sustained proximity to one's baby. The very matrix of our ability to love and bond in later life, maternal sensitivity – or lack thereof – also determines cultural tenor. Throughout history, the most brutal cultures have always been distinguished by maternal-infant separation. And yet how can maternal sensitivity develop when we effectively bully mothers into returning to the workforce before their uteri have even had time to shrink? This bullying takes various forms, from shaming – some of it disguised as concern ("Aren't you worried that you'll lose your place on the ladder?"); some of it indirect ("What's your post-baby body plan?") – to financial manipulation ("Surely you want your child to have the best?").

Two working mothers I knew – warm, vital, exhausted – were discussing mothering children under five. "I feel terrible admitting this," one exclaimed, "but looking after the children just isn't *enough*." Intrigued, I asked if she felt that motherhood was in itself insufficiently stimulating or whether she felt dispirited by the social response to motherhood. My question surprised her, and she paused. "Everyone thinks you're *boring* if you talk about children," she savagely said.

In *Erin Brockovich*, the 2000 biographical film that won Julia Roberts an Academy Award for Best Actress, the protagonist, a harried, working-class single mother of three, is asked why she won't quit her improbably demanding job. "How can you ask me to do that?" she asks. "This job – for the first time in my life, I got people respecting me. Up in Hinkley, I walk into a room and everyone shuts up just to hear what I got to say. I never had that. Ever. Don't ask me to give it up."

American director Brad Bird concurred with this damning analysis. Of the reaction to his editor wife's decision to dedicate herself to their children, he recalled: "When you're talking about work, everyone could connect with that – everyone GOT it, but once she said she was a mother, that she worked in the house, their eyes glazed over, and they kind of dismissed what she did."

Such dismissals are a form of bullying with which all mothers are familiar. Intimidated, we reframe our vulnerability into socially acceptable formats. Under the heading, "When is it appropriate to leave newborn to return to work?" a frightened new mother implored the internet: "The thought of it makes me want to cry my eyes out, but I can't take any more depending on my hubby and family for everything! It makes me feel completely miserable! I was always the type of girl to work for her money so I could buy what I want without anyone telling me otherwise!"

Using money as a metaphor for mastery over her world – the postpartum body is also a popular metaphor – this woman reached out to a universe of similarly overwhelmed strangers to no avail. What she really needed was tenderness and guidance to help her connect with her baby; what she got was glib replies about women easily leaving newborns and emotionally frozen complaints about "boredom".

At the most vulnerable time of their lives, mothers are repeatedly failed by the community.

The post-partum confinement period – a 30 to 40 day tradition throughout China, Greece, India, Japan, South Korea and Vietnam – is necessary not only to allow mothers to recuperate from the almost incomprehensible energetic expenditure that giving birth to a child entails, but to adjust to motherhood at a pace conducive to maternal-infant bonding. Hurried through the process – often in the unfamiliar environs of a hospital – women in their millions are failing to give birth without intervention and to breastfeed. The magnitude of the childbirth experience has been minimized for economic purposes, blighting an experience that could otherwise be infused with the purest bliss.

Our cultural de-emphasising of joy and pleasure in relation to the maternal–infant bond has numerous ramifications. As the relationship that determines our ability to accept ourselves in all of our flawed humanity is weakened, so is our ability to accept others in theirs; in that, a lessening of our capacity to love and to be loved. For what is the unhurried love of a mother if not complete acceptance of our ineptitude, of our fragility? Only maternal love can create that sense of security.

Michel Odent, the architect of water births, believes that our oxytocin system – oxytocin being the hormone of love, fundamental to birth and bonding throughout life – is growing weaker, and with catastrophic results. Our culture has come to be defined by adrenaline. In every area of our lives, we are jump-started, from the way in which we awaken (strong coffee, blaring alarms, television, radio) to the way in which we mate (Tinder, Grindr, Blendr, Tingle and so on).

But babies cannot be jump-started, and therein lies the fracture.

The Google doctrine stipulates that, "[f]ast is better than slow," but the veneration of acceleration is one of the greatest obstacles to intimacy and, perhaps, the most toxic in terms of parenting. An accelerated existence not only allows no time to consider either priorities or choices, but precludes deeply caring about those priorities or choices. Life just comes at us, and we react. The bar is now set by technology: jarring, bright, near-instantaneous. Intimacy, on the other hand, is quiet, slow

Attachment is the sum of repeated exposure, vulnerability, the consolidation of trust. There is no expediting love. And it is precisely at this point that our culture has started to fall apart. The fact that there is a need to specify attachment in relation to parenting tells us everything we need to know about the rupture between twenty-first century man and his heart. Emotion is no longer placed at the centre of human identity, which puts the very value of humanity at risk.

Professor Bruce Perry, the renowned child mental health researcher, stated that the most important property of humankind is the capacity to form and maintain relationships, which he sees as "absolutely necessary for any of us to survive, learn, work, love and procreate." This capacity is, he carefully explained, "related to the organization and functioning of specific parts of the human brain. Just as the brain allows us to see, smell, taste, think, talk and move, it is the organ that allows us to love – or not. The systems in the human brain that allow us to form and maintain emotional relationships develop during infancy and the first years of life."

Researcher David Metler agreed, finding that while there are almost no universal theories in Human Development and Family Studies as each depends on context and culture, there is something "very special" about attachment theory: supported by a substantial number of important empirical studies across various cultures and contexts, "the theory seems universal for humans."

In essence, attachment theory began taking shape during the Second World War, when Anna Freud, the founder of psychoanalytic child psychology (and Sigmund's daughter), observed that children who had been separated from their families for safe-keeping during the Blitz were suffering developmental issues. Despite the sometimes superior physical and intellectual ministering they received, these children were subject to fits of aggression, emotional withdrawal, head-banging, bed-wetting and soiling, tantrums, regression and other behavioural disturbances. They were, Freud realized, reacting to the disruption of their attachments, and she wrote movingly of the lack of adult appreciation for "the depth and seriousness of this grief of a small child."

Freud laid the groundwork for psychiatrist John Bowlby's exploration of the issue. In 1951, Bowlby, now known as the father of attachment theory, changed the landscape of developmental psychology with his powerful monograph for the World Health Organisation. In it, he emphasized that it is "essential" for the mental health of the infant and young child to "experience a warm, intimate and continuous relationship with his mother (or permanent mother-substitute) in which both find satisfaction and enjoyment. Given this relationship, the emotions of anxiety and guilt, which in excess characterize mental illness, will develop in a moderate and organized way."

In short: Germaine Greer's assertion that "[b]ringing up children is not a real occupation, because children come up just the same, brought up or not" could not be further from the truth. Parental devotion has an irreversible impact on children. Only 20 to 25 per cent of the brain is complete at birth, and even then, only in terms of autonomic function (heart rate, breathing, etc.); the rest of the brain is literally formed by the infant's experience of love or by its absence. Newborns have been shown to be so vulnerable that they are now referred to as "external foetuses"; in evolutionary terms, this allows babies to be "customized" to enable adaptation to their environment and circumstance. The first three years of life in particular are critical in terms of shaping both the capacity to form loving relationships in adulthood and the stability that makes happiness possible.

"Empathy, caring, sharing, inhibition of aggression, capacity to love and a host of other characteristics of a healthy, happy and productive person are related to the core attachment capabilities, which are formed in infancy and early childhood," Perry noted.

Given that this is the case, the current epidemic of disconnection makes it clear that our current child-rearing methods do not equip us with the capacity to sustain intimacy.

Certain biochemical systems – the stress response and emotional systems among them – can be set in what psychotherapist Sue Gerhardt describes as "an unhelpful way" if a child's early experiences of care-giving are inconsistent, insensitive or indifferent. Gerhardt added, "Even the growth of the brain itself, which is growing at its most rapid rate in the first year and a half, may not progress adequately if the baby doesn't have the right conditions to develop."

To be abandoned by mother in infancy – the neonatal brain is wired by evolution to interpret being left even only briefly as abandonment – not only damages our ability to connect with others (expression of need equals abandonment), but creates the sense of self-loathing that can destroy a life (through substance abuse, depression, anxiety disorders). Concomitantly, the World Health Organization reported that suicide rates have increased by 60 per cent since 1945.

In such a climate, is it surprising that the American Academy of Facial Plastic and Reconstructive Surgery found that the rate of face-lifts – the reconstruction of the identity we present to the world – has increased by 50 per cent? The media has been the fall guy for what is really a First World epidemic of self-loathing.

When mothers find themselves in the suburbs, isolated from status – and from partners forced to work hours historian Stephanie Coontz describes as "insane" – they can feel as if they're drowning. Because effective mothering requires not only a sustained investment of energy into the child by the mother, but an equal investment of energy into the mother by her partner, family and community.

The change we need demands a revision of priorities. We need to decide what constitutes a good life, and then adjust our lives – and policies – accordingly. As palliative care worker Bronnie Ware noted, one of the top five regrets of the dying is working too hard ("[People realize that they] missed their children's youth"). To achieve change, we need to start at the beginning. We need to rally around mothers on an individual and a cultural level, enabling them to bond with their babies so that the next generation does not suffer the wounds that have made ours so dysfunctional. Maternal vulnerability is neither indolence nor a sexist myth, but a normal response to our most sacred duty. Critically, we need to redefine our understanding of importance to include love, and to understand that far from being drudges, mothers are, in fact, creating the very tenor of our future.

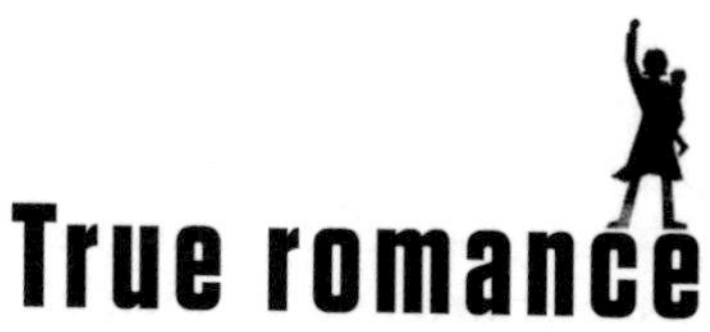

True romance

What love means

I had not slept for staring at my child,
for in herself, she was the dawn.

Up until I asked my husband about the most romantic moment in his life, I'd never really considered the issue. I was just curious, I think, in the way that every woman sometimes is for a glimpse into the internal world of the man with whom she shares her life.

"When we had Monkey", he said. "The first three years".

His reply shocked me. I had expected a resurrection of preadolescent ardour or thwarted love. But when he, in turn, asked the same question, I could think of no period that even approached the disorientating rapture of those years, a time often presented as an exodus from selfhood, a kind of hazing, or rite of initiation: something to be endured.

Together, we remembered my being wheeled to the maternity ward with our jaundiced baby after seventeen racking hours of labour, a rogue cannula that broke loose and splashed my face with blood, two and a half epidurals, morphine-induced nausea, second-degree internal tearing, and a sustained asthma attack on first standing. I was wheeled past trees laden with baubles – it was the night after Christmas – and into a new universe that defied every law. My husband and I were warned that mine was the experience of birth associated with impaired attachment and postnatal depression. In combination with my family history, it didn't look good.

The possibility no professional volunteered was that through parenthood, my husband and I would experience the kind of romance that, for years, endured as bliss.

In etymological terms, the roots of the word romance lie with the concept of chivalric adventure, and this was also my understanding: as a stylised distraction or escape spurred by disconnection. I subscribed to the notion of high romance – to the same picaresque instincts and exaggerated emotional investment responsible for the enduring popularity of Romeo and Juliet, Pride and Prejudice and the controversial Lolita; to the same reckless abandonment of self-consciousness facilitated by opiates. Poetry, which is implicit in romance, was the counterpoint to an existence that lurched from crisis to duty.

The poetic gesture was, to me, essential; the feeling behind it, less so. Even now, I find myself grading adolescent infatuations on the basis of their ability to make a lyrical experience of life – the boy who pressed that poem by Rilke into my fist as I disembarked from the school bus; the man who kissed me as 'Coney Island Baby' played, spring rain falling on the magnolia petals in the grass outside; that droll and modest lover who, in a black frock coat, walked with me most every day through the barley fields outside Oxford.

These and other recollections are the stars by which I navigate my past and, like stars, their light continues long after love's extinction. The boy who copied Rilke was expelled, and we lost touch. The Lou Reed fan became violent, necessitating police intervention. And, in the same way water is strained through muslin, the man in the black frock coat left my life.

The memory of their faces shimmers, but the magic was transient.

In my twenties, this blueprint was altered. The need for poetry was replaced by a need for validation. I had suffered a series of severe personal setbacks, and the resulting chaos rendered me indifferent to starlight. As if drowning, I grappled, seeking buoyancy, for the material. Sublime lawns and silks, Parisian lingerie, diamonds from Tiffany's: charged with status, each offering was an endorsement of value rather than feeling. For a girl who never once felt beautiful, it was intoxicating; otherwise, it meant nothing. Like gold stolen from mermaids in fairytales, it all turned to ashes in my hands. Mostly, I gave it away. I let a first-class return ticket to a distant city expire. I didn't care. My interactions were almost exclusively with a mirror. It was all about the perfect shoe, the perfect lipstick, the perfect hair; men were superfluous. The narrative of my life was mine alone.

As the vogue for romantic love accelerated with the emergence of the novel, romantic love was associated not only with the shaping of a woman's life into a narrative, but with liberation and self-realisation. Catherine Earnshaw, released from marriage to Edgar Linton and propriety by her desperate longing for the wilder Heathcliff; the expansion of Jane Eyre's narrow universe through the austere devotion of Edward Rochester. These archetypes are still in use – notably *Fifty Shades of Grey*'s phenomenon of knife-edge sexual torment, Christian Grey, and *Twilight*'s contained but lethal Edward Cullen. Romantic love still symbolizes a mule kick against the ascendancy of reason, that very modern god inured against what one writer called "the arbitrary rule of mysticism".

This human need for mysticism – surrender to an unknown truth, union – stands at the helm of all romantic feeling. It is, in essence, the same intimacy known in a mother's arms; in those who are deprived of the experience, the need freezes and, distorted, it can rent a life. All addiction has as its foundation skewed yearning for the same transcendence. For me, the spell of the material was broken by my brother's death; after his suicide, all I wanted was the renewal of my connection to the intangible.

Thus stripped back, I met the man who would, years later, become my husband. Without expectation or desire, he watched me grieve, and then adjust to life as the sister of a man who no longer existed. It was a long process, and he was only ever supportive. Others noticed the intensity of our attachment before we did. "Whenever you two are in the same room, it's as if no-one else is there", a friend of his complained. I was surprised by the observation, and repudiated it. My awareness of the attraction was checked by reluctance; he was the son of another friend, and I had no interest in further uproar.

Eventually, I capitulated – a decision that in the beginning others failed to understand. For me, that which set him apart was the unbroken focus of his intent. My husband is the only man I have ever known who is oblivious to interruption; he desires without ornament or gaiety, and was indifferent to the difficulties presented by our union. In certain respects it was, for me, a return to poetic, picaresque form. But the birth of our daughter changed everything; romance was no longer the stuff of gesture, but connection.

I became aware of the shift as I watched my daughter marvel at her first dawn. This was, hands down, the most exquisite moment of my life. She lay on her side, turned to the floury sunlight seeping in between the blinds, entirely still: she was entranced. "And this is morning", I whispered, so softly that I wasn't even certain I had spoken. Six hundred years before Christ, Sappho wrote:

> *Some say an army of horsemen, or infantry,*
> *a fleet of ships is the fairest thing*
> *On the face of the black earth, but I say*
> *It's what one loves.*
> *I had not slept for staring at my child, for in herself,*
> *she was the dawn.*

My handsome husband and I didn't make love for almost six months. I was enraptured, lost to my old life, and, in this obsession, disregarded author Ayelet Waldman – who famously wrote of her "smug well-being" and "always vital, even torrid" sex life in the wake of childbirth: I ignored my husband as a man. Instead, I revelled in him as a different thing altogether, far more seductive and important, and infinitely more resonant. My husband was no longer just a man: he was the father of my child. We watched each other evolve into parents, with all the fear, rage and confusion evolution can involve. Our eight-year-old is the incarnation of our union; we are forever fused by her blood. My old take on romance seemed vaguely ludicrous, as affected as a pair of spats. I no longer saw the point in "getting back to normal", that pantomime of pretending nothing had changed; I wanted to evolve from sexual posturing into a deeper consciousness: that of love.

Delirious as it can be, sex is only one kind of intimacy, and yet has become the cultural catchment area for all kinds of needs because our understanding of intimacy is so poor.

Brutal work schedules, related geographic isolation, and the concomitant fracturing of families has meant that there is little time for intimacy, and even less to teach the necessary skills. But intimacy, the axis of romance, is slow, based on the sharing of a life rather than show. In terms of intimacy, folding laundry together or sharing the feeding of a child can have more impact than the most extravagant bouquet. This basic human need for closeness is frequently mistranslated as a vital – even torrid – desire for sex, and not just because sexual interaction seems somehow more adult and less time-consuming; it simply does not necessitate the same enmeshment of vulnerabilities.

In the revised framework of early parenthood, there was, for us, all the liberation and self-actualization of traditional romance, and, more importantly, the honouring of connection. This magic was not transient. The sense was not of treasures pilfered, nor was it founded on glamour. In its place, a feeling of plainness and honesty, of life boiled to its bones, and in that, a joyous discarding of all elaboration. For once, life was enough. I have seen the same disregard of the world in those who become caretakers to a beloved.

The romantic gestures of my adolescence are no less charming because of the evanescent nature of the relationships that spawned them, and nor are the voyages and roses of my twenties less spectacular because they ultimately failed to fulfil. Both are like snatches of music sometimes heard in the distance, all the more beautiful for their remove. Each one is associated with a state or situation I needed to escape – the picaresque romantic adventure as saviour – but I no longer need liberating from my life.

There is, instead, promise, renewal. Beginning is its own romance. My husband and I remain bewitched by the sometimes stunning tumult of adaptation marriage entails; there is an alchemy in devotion we find irresistible. Everything else feels like practice.

The art of birth

An interview with Sheila Kitzinger

Birth is about entering into life jubilantly. Fully. And giving yourself to life.

In person, the eighty-five-year-old British author and anthropologist Sheila Kitzinger, once described as the "many-breasted Artemis, Goddess of Fertility", is radiant. In a hot pink and midnight blue silk, gilt-edged Chinese-style jacket decorated with tassels, she still dominates the room. She has always presented herself as a kind of exotic bird, favouring wild plumes of colour, texture and design. Crackling with intelligence and passion, she also demonstrates an intransigence at odds with her eccentric, informal persona (during one appearance, she was photographed on a table with her knees on her breasts – she was wearing a dress – in an effort to illustrate how one should not give birth).

One of the highest-profile natural childbirth activists in the world and the mother of five home-birthed daughters (her grandchildren were all birthed in water pools in her presence), Kitzinger lectures in midwifery at the Wolfson School of Health Sciences, England, is an honorary professor at Thames Valley University, campaigns unflaggingly for choice in childbirth, and is still a presence at birth rights rallies. Her workshop topics vary from complicated birth experiences to breastfeeding and the social anthropology of birth, and her twenty-three books, universally regarded as superb resources, include *Birth Crisis*; *Understanding Your Crying Baby*; *Birth Your Way: Choosing Birth at Home or in a Birth Centre*; and the perennial bestseller, *The New Pregnancy & Childbirth – Choices & Challenges.*

The scourge of reactionary obstetricians, Kitzinger introduced words such as “ecstatic”, “thrilling” and “dramatic” in relation to labour and birth. She reviles routine episiotomies and has reported that consistent prenatal support (from a midwife or doula) is associated with less pharmacological intervention, fewer instrumental deliveries, fewer c-sections, superior Apgar scores, less perineal trauma, more likelihood of breastfeeding at six weeks, and significantly lower rates of maternal depression. “Because birth is treated as high risk”, she has pointed out, “it often becomes high risk”.

Her work with mothers traumatized by birth is superlative (one in twenty mothers suffers PTSD). Kitzinger believes that many women who feel distressed after being disempowered during their child’s birth are wrongly muffled by antidepressants; what they really need, she says, is information and understanding. She even makes herself available through the Birth Crisis Network.

The Experience of Childbirth, her first book, was written after the birth of her fourth child in 1962. Barbaric practices such as episiotomies, enemas and forcing women to give birth on their backs were then routine and, as one writer noted, Kitzinger is largely credited with disabling the perfunctory administration of such practices. But, like Queen Victoria, Kitzinger refuses to acknowledge certain truths – that women may be accountable for bad decisions, say, or that some mothers are consciously cruel or indifferent; in her world, women are ever blameless, and those who err are simply wronged by men and “society”.

“I don’t know how useful it is to tell mothers they’re doing a bad job”, she primly announces as she seats herself in the hotel restaurant. “But if they’re doing a bad job, leave them! You don’t have to change them! I encourage analysis, but would not use that word with a woman; I’d describe it to her as a process.”

This infantilization of women is both obnoxious and disempowering, and detracts from the importance of her work. Historian Stephanie Coontz noted that such attitudes date back to early nineteenth century England, when the purity of women was emphasized as a reaction to the earlier perception of them as vulnerable to moral error.

When I note that some women actively choose to become masculinized in terms of sexuality and notions of value, Kitzinger bridles. "It's been foisted on us", she insists. "It really has been foisted on us. Certain behaviours are inculcated by society. I'm not talking just about men. I think women don't often realize they're making choices. We just drift into things because other people around us are doing it and it's accepted."

When I point out that drifting, too, is a choice, her smile tightens.

Other than when promoting women as the eternal victims of the patriarchy, Kitzinger can be riveting. One of her most acute observations is that the increasing medicalization – or industrialization – of birth has led to a widespread loss of confidence in women regarding their ability to give birth, and she has written about its impact on mothering.

"Women", she explains, "have certainly lost confidence with birth – but, mind you, read a bit of history. Birth was once a terrifying experience for women in which they prepared for death, because it was a very real possibility that they would die! They used to write letters of farewell, things like this. Women have not been confident in birth for a long, long time; but, on the other hand, they have been confident that they would get woman-to-woman support, and that changed when male doctors took over childbirth."

Kitzinger believes that this confidence can only be regained through the sharing of practical experience. "So it is very important", she says, "for those who have been through birth – and, indeed, other things – experience of sex, too – to talk about it in such a way that other women can make decisions. Oh, gosh – I didn't realize that it could be like this!" Momentarily, she abandons fastidiousness for humour. "We talk about sex as if it were exclusively a matter of a penis pushing into a vagina. Which is ludicrous! There are so many other aspects of sex as a positive physical experience – and even the sensual aspect of having a baby, you know?" Here she closes her eyes and visibly drifts into a kind of sensual trance. "Having a baby at the breast, cuddling a baby, breathing in a baby's essence, looking into a baby's big eyes ..." She blinks. "All that seems to me to be an aspect of women's sensuality which we ought to be celebrating."

Like many of those who work with women outside the medical sphere, Kitzinger has a deep sense of the holistic – that is to say, the whole picture: emotional, intellectual, physical and spiritual. "For example", she says, "when women opt for elective caesarean sections they are deliberately blanking out an experience. Now, maybe it's an experience they feel they have to blank out – and if so, I respect their choice … provided they know the side effects of caesarean sections on themselves and their babies, and on any subsequent pregnancy. But electing to have a caesarean section does mean saying: 'I'm not going to feel this', or: 'I'm going to numb myself to this.'"

Similarly, her views on breastfeeding are informed by an awareness of repercussions when the need for attachment is frustrated. "Your breast gives comfort, not only nourishment", she writes in *Understanding Your Crying Baby*. "Adults can feel comforted by seeing someone they love is in the room or by holding hands. This isn't so for a three-month-old baby. To feel completely secure the baby needs a closer clasp, more intimate contact, and to learn through the feel of the breast drawn into her mouth that all is well."

"Women often do have problems breastfeeding and find they can't breastfeed because they've already decided – and I know this for a fact – that they don't want the intense physical experience", she says. "Because breastfeeding is an intense physical experience. It may not be easy to get into, and it may hurt at first, but the satisfaction of responding to your baby instead of mechanically pushing a nipple in – *Open yer mouth! Get it in! Clamp it down! Get the baby on properly!* – is inestimable."

She exhales. "Well, of course, you do need to get the baby on properly, but you don't do that by force or by holding the back of a baby's head and shoving it onto the breast. I had my first baby in France, and was supposed to choose between a Catholic nursing home and a Jewish nursing home. In fact, I had my baby at home because neither of them seemed entirely satisfactory. But in the Catholic nursing home, not only did they have a picture of Christ on the cross, bleeding heavily, right opposite the delivery table, but I actually was with a woman and her new baby who was being shown how to breastfeed. A nun came to the door with the baby cocooned tightly, like one of those sweets, and she said, 'Steel yourself, Mother!' And then ran to the mother's naked breast and clamped the baby on. And that was showing the mother how to breastfeed."

Kitzinger's voice is thin and regal, and she punctuates announcements with a lightly arched brow. "Having a child is a maturing process", she gravely says. "And you grow up with it. And as the child grows, you grow more and more. And it eventually occurs to you that motherhood itself is educational! Education is not just something you do at a school desk. That said, I don't think you have to have a baby to be a woman."

Intently, Kitzinger explains that her fascination with womanhood and birth practice was triggered by her mother, a midwife. "She was a midwife before professional midwifery was recognized, and, in fact, when registrations started in Britain, Mother decided not to register. I suppose she didn't really see it as an academic subject. She'd started [nursing] when she was fifteen, and wanted to care for wounded soldiers – this was the end of the 1914–18 war. So she had, I think, a year in hospital with soldiers, and then a couple of GPs who knew the family asked if she would work with them while women were giving birth. Everyone had home births then. So she started working as a maternity nurse, and became a midwife." Her voice drops. "We were very close."

When asked what she learned about mothering from her mother, Kitzinger changes, and a slight speech impediment becomes obvious. "Oh, fweedom!" she exclaims, all eyes. "She allowed me a lot of fweedom, she really did. I became a vegetarian at the age of nine. I had an unusual childhood in the sense that my first memories are of going to mass pacifist meetings, and of resisting war, and of posters, and of famous pacifists like Dick Sheppard (Hugh Richard Lawrie Sheppard, founder of the Peace Pledge Union), who was the priest at St Martin in the Fields in London, and of course Gandhi was Mother's hero, so I grew up with all that. Very radical. Yes. And so when I had to decide between doing university work and letting my life open out a bit more, I didn't take the standard route. I had my five children. And I'm very glad I did."

She believes that Western women can be detached from their children because independence is promoted above intimacy. "Much of what we see in the media is about being independent, about going back to 'normal' after having a baby – as if you could go back to normality, instead of moving toward it. And there really is the feeling that power resides in keeping utter, utter control of one's whole life."

Kitzinger believes that the balance of power is changing, but slowly. "We are not going to change it overnight", she shrugs. "Women also need to talk about life in terms of pleasure and joy, and we really don't enough. We talk about power and fulfilment, about satisfaction in life as if it were a matter of getting to a particular grade in a particular job, of passing exams, and life isn't like that, really. We need to have a sensuous enjoyment of life, too. And if we don't have that, the rewards are very few. I believe that if you centre down in yourself, if you give yourself time for thought – meditation, reflection – to consider your place in society, your level of fulfilment, the fulfilment of others, and the big issue of rights, you can enter a space which enriches your experience of life."

In part, maternal desensitization can be attributed to the increasing presence of women in the corporate world, in which desensitization is promoted as an advantage. Psychologist Nichola Bedos recently noted that the women who seem to have the most difficulty with motherhood are those from the corporate sector, because their lives are about control. The children of such women, she observed, are rarely allowed to come first, and every aspect of the child's life is controlled: the mothers struggle to foist things upon their children rather than allowing their children to evolve.

The concept of "controlled crying" is an extension of this mania for control, and one that is, ultimately, emotionally dangerous for children. In *The Science of Parenting*, Dr Margot Sunderland examines the impact of depriving babies of comfort, and the news is bad.

"We haven't really registered all the dangers of controlled crying", Kitzinger agrees. "All these efforts to control babies have long-term effects – they're bound to! And it's not really 'controlled' crying, of course; it's uncontrolled crying, because the child has no control." Her voice softens. "The baby cries, and nobody comes. There's no response! What the baby actually learns is that other people don't respond."

In *Understanding Your Crying Baby*, Kitzinger elaborates

on the relationship between maternal stress and anxious babies, citing research findings that 60 per cent of women with excessively crying babies had a stressful pregnancy complicated by major life events.

"It may also be", she adds, "that when [a mother] has been made very anxious during pregnancy, she tends to be more anxious in her interaction with the baby, too, and assumes that the baby's crying is evidence of her failure in mothering. This leads to increased tension for both mother and baby, each acting on the other to trigger further frustration."

Birth, Kitzinger maintains, is an act of love. "Oh, birth is all about love!" she cries. "Birth is about feeling with your whole body, not just things happening in your uterus and vagina. It's about entering into life jubilantly. Fully. And giving yourself to life – love is about giving – and opening yourself to life. I have done research among midwives in traditional culture, and asked what they believe to be the most important thing. The answer – over and over again, in different languages – is to *free* her."

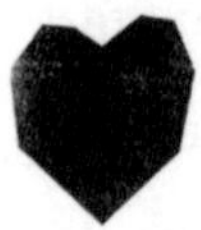

Chasing the Dragon

A love story in two parts

I sang so loudly – and spontaneously – that I startled myself, songs about tomatoes and nappies, potatoes and babies, butterflies and cows.

At eight months, Bethesda began to lurch face-first into my cleavage with a roar and, once she had inhaled the rich maternal perfumes of my breasts, literally shivered with anticipation. I laughed the first few times she did this – it was so artless, and so honest and so funny – but then I began to wonder – in the literal sense, to experience wonder – at her relationship with my body, a body with which I had only recently (and uncertainly) made peace, and at the intense intimacy breastfeeding had forged between us.

When she hadn't nursed for a few hours, I'd catch her glancing at my breasts with a covetous glint, or she would pat them with a plump little pink hand, or look up at me with big upslanted eyes as layered as the finest silt (carbon, moss, sand, mica) and say (tenderly, carefully): "*Na-na.*" This was her word for nursing, close enough to Mama, a word she knew and accurately used, but also far enough to distinguish a different level of experience. Mama was, my husband Alexander observed, her entire universe – I may as well have had my own private meteor showers and constellations, as I was both abstract and abstracted by the business of being a universe – but na-na was personal. Na-na was what happened between her and me, the language in which we communicated the miraculous nature of our relationship: *our thing.*

At first, I wasn't even sure I could do it.

My breasts, never small, became unmanageable during pregnancy. A walking Henry Moore sculpture, I could no longer cope without a brassiere at night. The weight of my breasts caused the straps to leave deep and aching grooves in my shoulders and I stooped, my back the crescent of the Man in the Moon (Isis is the goddess of moon and motherhood). I found it impossible to imagine those monsters as the source of anything but muscle spasms. And yet less than half an hour after her birth, Bethesda left two tiny love bites on my breasts, and then nursed like the angel for which she was named. An act that had, before her birth, seemed vaguely obscene – this perspective a legacy of my mother's emotionally dislocated parenting – was by her face reframed: nursing her felt like the most natural and uncomplicated thing in the world.

She fed like a dragon. We didn't leave our flat at all during the first six weeks. Bethesda was born during the hottest summer on record, so purdah wasn't such a stretch. We would lie in bed together all day, reading, cuddling, nursing; I had bought hand-stitched voile sheets in snow and cream and wheat. Muslin drapes fluttered at the open windows. Of all things, a cupcake shop was being fitted next door. Alexander wrote in the other room and took care of the housework.

Never in my life had I been so happy. I sang so loudly – and spontaneously – that I startled myself, songs about tomatoes and nappies, potatoes and babies, butterflies and cows. Inexplicably, the "Banana Boat Song" was Bethesda's favourite lullaby ("Work all night on a drink of rum/ Daylight come and me want to go home"), closely followed by recordings of David Bowie's "Golden Years" and Warren Zevon's "Werewolves of London". Alexander danced with her around the living room.

As she slept with us from the beginning (between me and the bolster against the wall; my husband sleeps like a corpse), we never had problems. We slept, she got the picture: night is for sleeping. Bethesda nursed as she slept, her face pale in the half-light from streetlamps outside.

Once she had finished, I would down two straight litres of water (during daylight hours, I drank four or more): I felt parched all day, every day. The texture of my breasts alternated between that of faceted granite and waterlogged brown paper bags. The locus of my fixity made me feel like a pervert.

Would that blocked milk-duct harden to mastitis? Why was my right breast twice the size of the left, which leaked in a way the right one never did? Would they hang like empty Christmas stockings after weaning? I walked around the flat like a refugee from a psychiatric ward – unwashed and with my hair unbrushed, one breast loose, in yesterday's pyjamas, intently muttering.

Feeding on demand meant that I never slept more than three consecutive hours for the first three months, and four consecutive hours for the next two. All new mothers are familiar with this torment. Micro-sleeps. Staring into space. Irritability, confusion, lapses in perception. And, finally, that increasing sense of depersonalization. My dreamscapes were fluorescent. Flying knives filmed at an oblique angle by a hand-held camera. The head of a doll rolling along a pavement. A baby dropped; my amplified horror. The psychotic imagery dissolved on waking, but still made me feel a little weird all day. But, as psychologist Bruno Bettelheim noted, scheduled feedings are disastrous as they reduce feeding to a mechanized procedure, and stop the baby associating her signals with satisfaction – in particular, satisfaction of her needs and of her ability to communicate her needs.

Bethesda rarely cried but when she did, it was because I had eaten something too complicated for her immature digestive system. Vegetarian sausages impregnated with garlic. Full cream milk. Chillies. And, most agonisingly for me, chocolate (the caffeine in it kept her up for hours). Who knew that colic was a myth conjured by doctors too embarrassed to admit they had no idea why newborns screamed? I cut out dairy, chocolate, spices. I mowed through protein – organic chicken, beef, fish, eggs – and brown rice, pasta, vegetables and fruit. My baby bloomed. She had been off the height and weight charts since birth. The sleep deprivation, the bland diet: all worth it.

"[H]ow beautifully designed the suckling of the baby at the mother's breast is", anthropologist Ashley Montagu wrote, "especially in the immediate postpartum period, to serve the most immediate needs of both, and from this to grow and develop in the service of all their reciprocal needs. What is established in the breastfeeding relationship constitutes the foundation for the development of all human relationships, and the communication the infant receives through the warmth of the mother's skin constitutes the first of the socializing experiences of his life."

My body was secondary to my daughter's. I was the chrysalis from which this butterfly emerged. I mourned the loss of my yoga silhouette, but also accepted that the plumpness of new mothers has a purpose: to cradle and warm our babies as they feed. I have always wanted one thing for her, and that is peace. Peace with herself, peace with the world.

Einstein believed that the most important question we can ask ourselves is whether we feel the world is a friendly place, and I agree; in the answer to that question lies the axis of our life philosophy. By continuing to keep Bethesda close, even though I have stopped breastfeeding, I make her feel secure, and because she feels secure, she is as merry and placid a child as I have ever seen. I want her to feel comfortable in her skin, because I never did in mine.

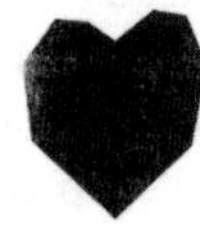

Let them eat cake

A conversation with Michelle Shearer

We feel undervalued because we are *undervalued.*

In February 2010, Michelle Shearer, the slight, tan, forty-year-old British-born founder of the collaborative consumption revolution MamaBake, was picking up her two children at school when, "out of the blue", a girlfriend gave her homemade lasagne. "That's the kind of person Bec is", Shearer explains, "always giving, always thinking of others". The two women had been to high school together, lost touch, and rediscovered each other on Facebook before finding that they had settled "up the road from one another" on the North Coast of New South Wales, Australia, where Shearer lives with three free-range parrots and her family in a "feral and chaotic" house. "Anyway", she continues, "the lasagne meant I didn't have to cook that evening, so I went surfing instead. Afterward, my mind started ticking over how I could reciprocate, and it occurred to me that the pressure to immediately reciprocate took away the joy of simply receiving." Shearer began to muse on the average mother's wariness of accepting any kind of help, particularly because to do so "suggests that one has bad days, so therefore no assistance needed, thank you very much!" Her thoughts then turned to communal cooking: mothers lightening the load for each other, swapping food, investing a little time, and making life easier. "I envisioned a tight community where we could be real with one another", she says. "And the children of MamaBakers learn about community. They learn firsthand about the power of humanity, of rolling up sleeves together and working – something kids don't see any more because parents scurry off to work. At MamaBake, women work together and their kids are in the mix – helping, cutting, kneading, stirring, being involved, participating. They learn about food, where it comes from, and how it can be prepared and cooked. They get to try new meals, new flavours, new styles of cuisine. They enjoy the wonderful social environment with other children and other mothers. Sharing, swapping, collaborating: all amazing human behaviours we have long ignored and dismissed." Shearer held the first MamaBake that month. Four women turned up, cooked one big-batch meal each, and at the end of the session the meals were divided among them. "It was", Shearer says, "so simple. We had family dinners for four nights: a eureka moment. From there, the group mushroomed each week until it had to split up into smaller groups. By April, I'd created a Facebook group to co-ordinate everyone." MamaBake now has over 20,000 likes on Facebook. MamaBake communities are internationally active. On the MamaBake website, the conversation alone is worth the price of admission. There are hundreds of inspired, wholesome big-batch recipes (the most downloaded is the cauliflower pizza base), first-person essays and forums. And it all evolved from the tender gesture of one woman to another.

AGB: There is a warmth and support in the MamaBake community that is mostly absent in more structured social situations for mothers. I love the humour and sincerity. That and the three-ingredient honey nut brittle that brought me and my husband to our knees – we ate the lot in an hour.

MS: The warmth and support is there because we created MamaBake to be the warmth and support we all need when we have children. Warmth and support are missing in our society. We have forgotten the value of community and love and care and kindness and neighbourliness in the pursuit of flat-screen televisions, big houses, cars, and stuff and more stuff … The bohemia of the 1960s morphed into navel-gazing narcissism where it is now all about exploring the self and radical self-love, which is all great, but I think we've gone overboard. Yes, we're individuals and yes, let's look after ourselves, but let's remember to look out for *one another*, too. We need to remember that we live in a world of other people; there's no better feeling than taking care of and considering others and being taken care of and considered. The balance is totally out of whack. Society's values are upside down and it's not serving anybody apart from the corporates. We're all paying the price in so many ways. I think we're now experiencing a backlash against that in the form of collaborative consumption and a gentle shift back to coming together that is being led by Generation Y folk.

AGB: One of the reasons my husband and I left the city was to escape the lack of sincerity. Everyone we knew was so stressed that they could barely function as members of a community. The levels of anxiety were cancerous. Crazy work schedules made recreation impossible; life outside work was all about stress relief rather than real pleasure or connection.

MS: Without real community, we shrivel and don't thrive so much. Together we can do so much more, be so much more.

AGB: I found myself experiencing an almost physical longing for the company of other mothers after the birth of my child.

MS: Most of us don't even realize that isolation is responsible for our sadness because we haven't ever known what it is to really be with other women – working alongside women, talking in depth with women, experiencing the daily grind with other women. I think the heartache manifests as mental illness, depression, anxiety and the like. We self-medicate with more "me-time" when what we need is more "we-time".

AGB: In part, I think that this is because women still feel lesser-than. This manifests in a mania for constant physical improvement, which requires an exorbitant investment – of time, of money, of energy. I mean, the level of narcissism is just staggering. And once a baby comes along, such self-involvement is no longer possible unless mothering is almost entirely delegated. So mothers who choose to actively mother are left with one option: to live in love, but relinquish all social value.

MS: We feel that we're without value because we are not valued. Where are we valued? Mothers are the invisible demographic. We are not held in high regard anywhere; we are ignored by society. Our work is undervalued. A young feminist said during a recent clash I had with her about feminism that we aren't going anywhere because all women want to do is get married and have kids! I know what she is saying – that we make ourselves more vulnerable by doing that – but she was also oblivious to the vast potential power held by women at home with children. No-one speaks of us, no-one calls on us, no-one asks us anything. We feel undervalued because we are undervalued.

AGB: I became an attachment parent on instinct, and not because I was following some branded movement: it just felt right to breastfeed on demand, to co-sleep, and so on. But the reactions! You'd think I'd joined the neo-Nazi party. It was suggested that I wanted to return to the 1950s; that I was some kind of privileged wife who could think of no better way to spend an afternoon than curling her daughter's hair; that I was right-wing, an evangelist, uninformed, and so on. Even though I'm mostly Buddhist. Even though we're mostly broke. Even though I'm married to a significantly younger man who does all the housework. And even though I was, until recently, the primary breadwinner. The only thing that mattered was dismissing views that made them feel uncomfortable. The big word on the table was "guilt". In this forum, guilt is the disqualifying agent. If one mother reacts with guilt to another mother's choices, there can be no measured discussion even if that discussion is necessary for the revision of cultural priorities. Never mind the recent neurobiological research backing every choice attachment parents make; to advocate attachment parenting is seen by certain factions as a gesture hostile to gender parity. What I don't get is why women who, after criticizing the patriarchal model on the basis of discrimination, then adopted it as their own – promoting a traditionally masculine definition of success, seeking a traditionally masculine idea of power and embracing pornography, a traditionally masculine spin on sexuality. Shying away from active motherhood and all that motherhood entails is only part of that.

MS: I don't think feminists quite knew – and still don't know – what to do with mothers. Here we are doing the baby thing with all our baby bits that we women have, and yet feminists just don't quite know what to do with it. The fact of the matter is in the vast majority of cases, when kids come along, we are suddenly thrown back to the 1950s of the worst kind, exposing society for what it is: UNequal. The women are at home and the men are at work – or both are at work – and guess who's still doing the lion's share of the domestics and the brain power that goes into the drudgery of it all? Women! Society doesn't know what to do with us. They prefer mothers to hop in and out of the economy as it suits them, paying us crappy wages. And the feminists would rather we just shut up and stayed nice and schtum. Silly move. Free mothers up, free them up to think, free them up from the domestics, stick them in a think tank with some social issues for a week, and see what happens! There needs to be a MotherThinkTank. That's my next project – once I've got all mothers some free time from MamaBaking, that is. There is so much potential power there. Silly feminists ignoring us mums. We should be revered! Mothers are doing this thing that, in other societies, is done together; our culture has set it up all wrong and here we are doing it, to the brink and back and only just hanging in there. What of the strength it takes to birth, to parent, to shoulder the burden of the domestics? Caring for all, thinking of all. And yet we remain ignored. Foolish, foolish!

AGB: At core, it's all about terror of subjugation, exploitation, powerlessness. Babies make you so vulnerable. What was it Shakespeare said about times of war? "Woe unto them that are with child, and to them that give suck in those days"? Or did Jesus say that? I think it may have been Jesus. At any rate, it was definitely not Groucho Marx. The bottom line is this: vulnerability can be terrifying. It's easier to pretend to be invulnerable and to avoid emotional enmeshment. There's less to lose.

MS: When we have children, no matter where we are on the path of self-evolution, we suddenly have to gather our values and put them out there in the way that we parent, for all the world to see. Wow, the world can be a brutal place for the new mum. We are so vulnerable. So many theories, textbooks and parenting gurus assuring us that theirs is "the right way"! It's dizzying. With no elder woman "compass" encouraging and guiding us as we journey along the path of motherhood, we constantly doubt ourselves. We think we see others doing it the right way and feel bad and guilty for not doing as well as Mrs Jones. And so we become overwhelmed, get lost, and forget to tune into what we innately know. We forget to back ourselves. I believe our vulnerability is directly linked to the nuclear family model, leading to the isolation and division of women at all stages of their lives.

AGB: The superwoman myth has a lot to answer for.

MS: Why do we perpetuate this myth that we're okay when we really are not? I think we've gotten our knickers in a right royal twist about seeming to be killing it when we're not. The MamaBake groups are so intimate, and working together in the way we do is a great leveller, so it is easier for a woman to say how it is to the others. All women have good days and bad days and to pretend that this isn't the case, to buy into that whole superwoman myth, is so destructive to women.

AGB: Why, as a community, do we need to make a fuss of new mothers?

MS: Because we need to focus on and value mothers as a whole. We are a long-ignored demographic in society, yet we are doing the most vital work for society. New mothers need to be supported through the long transition of early motherhood, and this can only happen properly through the women around her who have been through it: seasoned mothers.

AGB: But the culture, too, needs to change its focus from what is really a kind of mindless industrialisation to what can be designed as an almost artisanal mindset: measured, skilled, respectful. Now, what should mothers do for other mothers who have just moved to the area?

MS: Make them welcome in a number of ways: knock on the door to say hello, offer help in some small way, invite them over for coffee to introduce them to friends, offer to show them around, answer questions about the area, give them your phone number.

AGB: And apply this to sick or overwhelmed mothers?

MS: Yes, because when we go down, the family goes down. So much rests on the mother thinking about the household and doing stuff for the household. She must be held and supported by other mothers so that she can recover and be well again. We all need to rally around sick mothers – leave meals on their doorsteps, do things that need doing. Working together and sharing experiences of motherhood builds trust and friendship among mothers and so allows for this kind of support, far more so than if we remain hunkered down within our own four walls, away from everyone. Generally, mothers struggle on and the sickness lingers, but no mother can thrive like this.

AGB: Absolutely. I've noticed that a lot of families of origin are either absent, hostile or uninterested, leaving parents completely marooned. In many cases, the only offers of help are financial. They're not available for emotional support because love and babies are not the priority. The *New York Times* ran an article about this called "When Grandma Can't Be Bothered". I engineered the estrangement from my own family of origin when Bethesda was four. They created unimaginable difficulties in our lives – in retrospect, it was almost improbable. Complete chaos.

MS: In Thatcher's England, there was no such thing as "society"; everything was about the individual. So those of us who grew up in the eighties saw lots of women leaving the family and the re-emergence of latchkey kids. The value of community was entirely lost – what a shame after whole countries pulled together after World War Two! So as kids got older, they moved away, or the parents moved away in pursuit of gain. Our mothers left to pursue the golden promise of a career. And as we watched our mothers pull away, it sent us a message around the world about the value and importance of family, and the state of families today reflects those actions. Certainly in my instance, anyway. My own mother always did well at school, and changing times meant that as a woman, she was able to get a degree and pursue a full-time career. For that I'm proud, but I also think we lost something in the process as a family and as individuals. And then I did it, too.

AGB: I couldn't wait to leave home. That era was toxic on so many levels. It was a social experiment: the divorce generation. So many children were messed up. Suicides everywhere.

MS: My nanna tells me that she just doesn't understand how people can leave their families. I moved to Australia with absolutely no idea of the consequences. I loved my family of origin then and I love my family of origin now, but back then it was all a big adventure: I was finally striking out alone! But while my little family here is thriving, my grandparents are in England up one end of the country, and my sisters are down the other. I was recently watching this dreadful hospital show where people end up in A&E – it's a reality TV thing, awful voyeuristic stuff – and one chap, an East Ender, a genuine Cockney, was brought in. When his family came to see how he was, they spoke in hushed whispers of "the family pulling together", and said that no matter what, "the family would be there". It moved me almost to tears because for me, growing up, my family wasn't my bedrock in that way, it was a troublesome and turbulent place. What greater gift is there to give our children than to let them know that no matter what, we're always there for them?

AGB: The only reason my mother never had a career is because my late father, a simultaneously anarchic and authoritarian Northern Italian, wouldn't allow it, but she always, always wanted to work. She was a very young mother, and never especially invested in mothering. My youngest brother was in boarding school by the age of ten or so, despite the fact that they lived in the same city. She's actually admitted that she just didn't "feel" what a mother should feel for her daughter. So I was very wary of becoming a mother, terrified that I, too, would just want to escape. The biggest shock was discovering that I revelled in the intimacy – all I wanted to do was kiss my baby and bake. Cake is a universal language. It certainly answers a lot of questions around here!

MS: Since Viking times, cakes have been given as a symbol of esteem. They would generally be made with refined sugar and nuts, which were then hugely expensive; the greater the expense, the greater the esteem. I don't think a huge amount has changed today. It's always very special when someone makes us a cake. My friend Bec always makes me some kind of heart-shaped cake when she comes over, and each time it invokes feelings of care. To me, a cake is a celebration of someone. I'm not that crash-hot at making cakes, but they still mean something – I've always tried to pull cakes together with good feelings in my heart, though the end result probably doesn't reflect those feelings. My cakes are usually a bit of a kerfuffle. In Pagan days, they used to roll cakes down hills to represent the motion of the sun or something, and that's about all my cakes are good for!

AGB: [laughing] Your first memory of cooking?

MS: Mum showing me a battered black, yellow and orange recipe book. She used it for all kinds of meals. I baked a Victoria Sponge from that book. I remember the smell of it, and how it would fall apart, and knowing how to hold it to keep it together long enough so I could read the recipe. Mum loved to cook exquisite thirteen-course French meals for dinner parties and experimented with vegetarian food, but wasn't into the day-to-day chore of cooking. Mostly, that was left to my stepfather, who was never afraid of good old English fare such as potatoes, dirty old sausages, beans and pies!

AGB: At core, what does cooking represent? In the grand sense, I mean.

MS: Well, that's it, really, isn't it? The core. Cooking is the heart of the family – it's what nourishes us and keeps us alive. And how we do that has consequences. As cooking and the serving of food is fundamental to human existence, it makes sense to honour that within the family. In cooking well, we honour the family. Whether our children grow and thrive depends on what we cook.

The MamaBake MamaFesto

MamaBake believes that through group big-batch baking, mothers can find themselves time-liberated to think, create, be and do whatever they like.

MamaBake encourages an atmosphere of trust and honesty in its in-real-life groups so that women feel free to share their real experience of motherhood.

MamaBakers judge not the woman for the state of her house; clean or chaotic.

MamaBakers take a "curiosity without judgment" approach to other mothers.

MamaBakers look out for one another and rally when needed.

MamaBakers are comfortable giving and receiving help when needed and know that this act in itself enables others to give and receive.

mamabake.com

The gift of femininity

Navigating gender

Life without femininity – devoid of mystery, emotion, gentleness and the unerring power of a woman's love – is no life at all.

As a child, I was entranced by the top drawer of my grandmother's dresser. In it were the gloves of her youth, another life: elbow-length white buttoned kid; cashmere-lined black leather; taupe silk; others. There were seamed stockings, too, and perfumes in frosted glass bottles, and tiny brass lip-colour compacts from the forties with their thick, sticky reds. Thirty years and the heat of another continent had not diffused their fragrance. Every object had retained its mystery – and not only from a historical perspective; each represented an aspect of femininity absent in my mother, with her jeans and bare, dry lips and razored shag.

The product of a generation with a very different understanding of womanhood, my mother was rarely tender. I remember crying bitterly as she hacked at my hair, but my tears had no effect. For years, I was called a boy by other children and by shopkeepers, who frequently remarked on my handsomeness. With an anguish that manifested as heat – I will never forget that unrefracted flush of shame – I implored her to buy me long, white-patterned nylon socks trimmed with lace, and wore them even when the lace grew tattered because they demarcated me as female.

To be a girl: that was the thing.

This phase was brief. In increments, it became obvious to me that femininity was old hat. My grandmother – compassionate, emotional, gentle – belonged to history.

The denigration of femininity was everywhere. Intelligent women were derided as unattractive; beautiful women were defamed as mindless; devoted women were mocked as bestial, inferior, hens. As Mick Jagger sang:

She's the worst thing in this world
Well, look at that stupid girl.
Shut up, shut up, shut up.

Love was no longer *au courant*. I watched as women, after decades of marriage, were jettisoned by the fathers of their children. Some descended into alcoholism; some neglected children to find themselves. "No whatever it was we had", American poet Anne Sexton wrote in 1969, "no sky, no month – just booze". Five years later, Sexton gassed herself wearing her mother's furs.

Our culture is now one of masculine triumphalism, in which transhistorically feminine expressions – empathy, sweetness, volubility, warmth – are seen as impediments to a woman's professional trajectory in many sectors. The market is awash with literature warning women of the perils of their femininity in the workplace. "Stop apologizing!" Lois Frankel cautions in *Nice Girls Don't Get the Corner Office*. In *How to Say it for Women*, Phyllis Mindell scolds women for "prefacing sentences with I think or I feel", making it clear that subjectivity – transhistorically, the feminine slant – is considered an attribute of losers. However specious, objectivity – a masculine conceit – must be feigned.

Accordingly, a number of women I know stifled their sensitivity and maternal instincts to compete in male-dominated spheres, eroding – and, often, destroying – the most important relationships of their lives. Talented women are now presented with only one model of fulfilment: career success and its concomitant remuneration. In *How Remarkable Women Lead*, Joanna Barsh, a happily married, successful career woman with healthy, high-achieving daughters, announces – with improbable earnestness – that she felt "invisible" on realizing that "[o]ther women surely had gone further, had done more". Visibility is conferred not by contentment but by the ratification of dispassionate authorities in this harsh universe. I was considered "gifted" at school not because I was emotionally literate, but because I am intelligent and intelligence is far more valuable in our culture despite the fact that value itself is predicated on emotion. The bar is masculine, and women must adopt traditionally masculine characteristics – cultivated insensitivity, goal-orientated thinking, the prioritizing of the material – to compete.

Anthropologist Sheila Kitzinger concurs, believing that women have, en masse, rejected the traditionally feminine acceptance of ever-shifting priorities in favour of the male idea that power resides in "keeping utter, utter control of one's whole life" – control of our bodies, control of our emotions. And yet the female body, understood as sacred through the mother goddesses of the Neolithic era, is generally unresponsive to attempts at control. When not hijacked by chemicals, our rhythms are governed by forces ranging from the affective to the lunar: emotional stress has as much of an impact on our ability to bear a child as any biological factor, which is why holistic fertility practitioners report successes where Western treatments fail. Physiologically, we are informed by mystery, and therein lies our potency.

Our sensitivity to forces outside the self is a gift.

I fought against this mutability, this responsiveness, throughout my adolescence and twenties. I did not want the hallmarks of a group forever associated with subjugation, of a gender so poorly represented in the arts. As critic Cyril Connolly wrote, "there is no more sombre enemy of good art than the pram in the hall", and author Erica Jong agreed, noting that the "queens of literature" – Austen, the Brontës, Woolf – were all childless.

To be a woman was, I felt, to be burdened with ambivalence, challenged by biological imperatives, torn. The slightest deviation in my menstrual cycle triggered panic. Because unlike men, we are reminded each month of our mortality, our potential. The unavoidable choices we make as a result can feel like burdens, or like questions we just don't feel like answering. Aged eleven when I began menstruating, I wanted none of it.

This aversion to femininity was not responsible for my

disordered relationship with food, but it was certainly a contributing factor. Puberty was, to me, a sledgehammer. I was appalled by the loss of control, humiliated by my breasts, and – appropriately – attempted to disguise them with my father's white cotton business shirts. The same shame of my childhood compromized my teens, if from the opposite pole: where I had once burned because my femininity was overlooked, I now burned because it was too overt. I missed the leanness of my girlhood, and the lack of judgement that such a body conferred.

Seeking control, I alternated between bulimia and an informal anorexia – informal because I never identified with anorectics as a group, nor did I ever weigh myself or seek starvation: I simply "forgot" to eat. My diet? Chocolate and low-tar cigarettes. Chinese food on occasion. White grapes, lychees, jelly, milk. I don't recall feeling especially hungry, but nor was I especially self-aware. The concern of friends was a constant. Detached, I loved the feeling of transparency, lightness, of independence from the material. And when I did remember to eat, I gorged and vomited so silently and swiftly that no dining companion ever knew. Emotionally, I was a ghost of sorts. Psychiatrists call it dissociation. Life was experienced at a distance, making it easy for me to "forget" to feel.

Sex, for me, was masculinized, a matter of goals (orgasm), stress relief and stimulation in place of connection. At times, I focused so exclusively on the mechanics of the act that my partner almost seemed incidental. In this respect, I was not alone. Women with insufficient feeling are, in the manner of jump-starting a car, now expected to compensate for a lack of connection, love or interest with pornography. Accustomed to self-objectification, an increasing number of women advocate the use of porn as a way of tolerating trivial sexual exchanges. If we stare intently enough at the screen, we don't have to confront the absence of intimacy with a partner. The experience thus assumes a virtual sheen and with that, a dilution of emotional importance: sex as recreation.

In 2011, journalist Rachel Olding wrote of privileged schoolgirls: "Theirs is a world in which giving a boy a blowjob in the toilets is 'pretty slutty' but you'll shrug it off the next day … Waking up not knowing where you are is not unusual." Such reductionism pivots on the understanding of sex as trivial, an understanding that is masculine in scope. The transhistorically feminine perception of sex as potentially life-altering – in terms of emotion and reproduction – once gave the act gravitas; the sensual and spiritual dimensions of sex are now in the process of being lost.

This disconnection between body and spirit is fatal in terms of intimacy, both with the self and others, and the resultant loneliness is reflected in the rates of substance use and abuse: in the United States alone, the number of women presented in states of life-threatening intoxication to ER rose by 52 per cent over a decade, and there has been a 400 per cent increase in the prescription of antidepressants, mostly to women. Historian Peter Wehrwein described the increases as "astounding". This disconnection also has permanent sexual repercussions: women are five times as likely to catch a sexually transmitted disease other than HIV than men (out of the 500,000 people diagnosed with a STI each day, over 400,000 are women). Certain feminists rebrand these tragedies as evidence of parity, but female biology is significantly more vulnerable to both substance abuse and sexual diseases than the male, sometimes to the point where women are rendered infertile.

Repudiating the vulnerability I felt had wrecked the lives of women around me, I modelled myself on my controlled father. I wanted his freedom and his focus. To him, a family was an aquarium: controlled, contained. To the women I knew, a family was everything. Consciously, the prospect of motherhood repelled me. Babies were boring, demanding, inarticulate. I scorned suggestions that I could be "missing out", observing that the charm of weddings and babies often palled, but professional success was forever.

And then I heard my daughter's cry.

On first hearing that little voice – as fine and friable, I felt, as cotton thread, the impact on my soul was that of the highest magnitude of earthquake, those that occur every hundred years, say, or every thousand. The old shell I called myself cracked and was swallowed by a sudden crevasse, and just as suddenly was lost in the commotion. That which I felt was not joy or even a willingness to throw myself in the path of a car to save her, but simply this: a desire to be with her so plunging I would have killed for it.

For the first time, my femininity was a requirement. That sense of being unbridled was intoxicating. I no longer had to feign disinterest. Feelings I'd stifled for decades could be expressed without censure or scorn. Kissing, nursing, coddling, caring: even in writing these words, I am aware of the perception of them as secondary to industry rather than as the hallmarks of a well-lived life. It is only through my daughter that I have come to realize that a life without femininity – devoid of mystery, emotion, gentleness and the unerring power of a woman's love – is no life at all. The kindnesses we deride as anachronistic, the affective scope dismissed as neurotic, the gentleness discouraged in our children lest they be earmarked as weak: these are expressions of humanity's best, the things that in the end, we will remember, unlike the dispassionate approval of a boss.

From the perspective of my peers, my grandmother was wasted – "gold put to the use of paving-stones", as Emily Brontë once wrote. Forced to leave school at twelve by an alcoholic father, she did not excel financially or professionally, and died before she grew old, in racking pain, having rejected every hand but mine. But to me, her successes were incomparable. She loved without reserve, enabling me to survive storms that felled others. "You are so blessed", she said, holding my face in her hands. Her femininity is the torch I now use to illuminate my daughter's path. Its light will burn through generations.

The cult of idleness

A different way to live

Doing nothing might just save the planet.
Dan Kieren, *The Book of Idle Pleasures*

In 2003, Gavin Pretor-Pinney and Tom Hodgkinson, then both thirty-five, agreed to celebrate the tenth anniversary of their magazine, *The Idler*, by taking a break for a few months, loafing about, living without a plan. Entirely self-funded and inspired by Dr Samuel Johnson's 1758 journal of the same name, *The Idler* had established itself as the organ of the highbrow slacker: erudite and elegantly designed, it was the British take on anti-consumerism, very, very funny, and featured contributors and interviewees such as artist Damien Hirst, philosopher Alain de Botton and novelist Will Self, who was once involved with Hodgkinson's wife. Appropriately, it made no profit; Hodgkinson and Pretor-Pinney earned their living through the graphic design commissions it inspired.

By then the father of two toddlers, Hodgkinson rented a farmhouse in rural Devon for six months, while Pretor-Pinney, a bachelor, swapped his London apartment for one in Rome. Hodgkinson fell in love with the farmhouse, where his wife later conceived their third child and where the family remains, and it was in Rome that Pretor-Pinney, idling over a cappuccino one morning, decided to form the Cloud Appreciation Society, a non-profit international organization dedicated to "fighting the banality of blue-sky thinking".

"Interestingly", Pretor-Pinney recalls, "there weren't many clouds in Rome, and I missed them; I missed the changing beauty that they brought to the sky. So many people have childhood memories that are evoked by clouds or reading about clouds. This impression is formed at a very vulnerable age, which means it's laid down quite deeply. And then, somehow, it becomes dormant. In Rome, I spent my days strolling around churches, gazing at baroque frescoes, noting that pretty much all the apostles reclined on the clouds as they surveyed the congregation below, crepuscular rays of sunlight bursting out behind their heads, symbolizing spirit. I always make a point of reminding people that clouds aren't something to complain about. They may be so mundane and everyday that we become blind to them, but that's not a reason to forget about their beauty."

The Cloud Appreciation Society now has close to 38,000 members in seventy-eight countries. It has inspired people of all ages to pause in the course of otherwise frantic lives. One decided to paint clouds on a burned-out car abandoned in his local woods; others have taken up cloud painting, writing, photography. Registering beauty, it seems, can change your life.

Had the society been founded by a more entrepreneurial individual, Pretor-Pinney muses, it would now be earning "pots of money. It could have been turned into a really, really successful business, and I haven't done that at all. You pay your four pounds, and that's life membership. I just wanted it to be easy – I didn't want to be taking money from people every year. And that's part of the appeal, I think; it's not at all commercial."

The organization's success had Pretor-Pinney wondering whether he should write a tribute to clouds, healing the damage done by inept geography teachers the world over. His agent loved it, but publishers were harder to convince; twenty-eight turned the gentle, lisping, balding, half-deaf cloud enthusiast down, citing difficulties in categorizing *The Cloudspotter's Guide* ("Is it, um, meteorology?"). Even the editor who published it initially rejected it, claiming to have been bullied by a resolutely blue-sky marketing department. "It was an incredible struggle to get it published", Pretor-Pinney marvels.

Described by one critic as the bible of a new religion, *The Cloudspotter's Guide*, ostensibly a love song to water particles but in actuality an ode to joy itself, sold over 250,000 copies and has been published in seventeen languages. Pretor-Pinney, who is prone to fits of giggling, immediately became a fixture at literary and rock music festivals, where he stood on stage pointing to slide presentations of clouds that resembled hearts, the Abominable Snowman, and six-legged pigs, and asked people to name them ("I don't mean give it a name – like 'Philip' – merely, identify its genus and species"). Demographics were transcended: boffins, stoners, children, the literati, suburbanites, the elderly and corporate men were uniformly dazzled by his open excitement.

"So after all that", Pretor-Pinney, now a married father-of-two, explains, "the publishers were like: 'What's your next book gonna be?!' Whereupon I rather impulsively said, 'Well, I think waves are rather interesting, but I'm afraid I don't have a book proposal.' And they were like: 'Don't worry – we'll write one!'"

To Pretor-Pinney's relief – he has always lacked literary confidence – *The Wavewatcher's Companion* was received with equal, if not greater, enthusiasm. "If you've ever wondered why your heart beats, snakes slither, suspension bridges collapse, butterfly wings shimmer, saucers fly, traffic jams – it's all about waves", he recites.

He first became intrigued by waves when he found himself glider-surfing the Morning Glory, a majestic, columnar, 1000-kilometre-long Australian cloud. Its similarity to an ocean wave, he noted, was startling. So Pretor-Pinney applied what he describes as his "Asperger's-like" focus to waves, discovering their connection to every other kind of wave – infrared, micro, shock, light, Mexican. Like its predecessor, *The Wavewatcher's Companion* achieves the improbable: it restores magic and meaning to the world for many. The fact that he is now recognized as one of the figureheads of the Slow Revolution surprises Pretor-Pinney, who only ever wished to be allowed to exist in a state of perpetual aesthetic rapture. A private man, he prefers rambling through the Somerset countryside to refining the new philosophy regarded by many as our culture's salvation.

Philosophically, the Slow Movement is not, as academics Wendy Parkins and Geoffrey Craig explain in their book *Slow Living*, about inertia, a return to the past ("pre-McDonald's

Arcadia"), or relocation to a picturesque Tuscan village, but "an attempt to live in the present in a meaningful, sustainable, thoughtful and pleasurable way".

This pursuit of conscious – and intelligent – deceleration is the new quest. Senior journalists the world over have called for the adoption of Slow Word, an ethical, measured, factually correct journalism to replace the destructive, scandal-triggered news cycle of what one writer described as "aggression, allegation and assertion".

Slow Reading, too, is a reaction to the religion of efficiency. "There is something similar between a reading method that focuses primarily on the bottom-line meaning of a story in a novel and the economic emphasis on the bottom line that makes automobile manufacturers speed up assembly lines", university press editor Lindsay Waters noted.

In the same vein, Slow Travel is all about following the easy, local rhythm of quiet villages, sleeping in medieval farmhouses and ambling through the countryside. Slow Architecture involves gradual construction and local building traditions (both of which are, curiously, ultimately more cost-effective than hit-and-run construction jobs). And Slow Money steers financiers to invest capital into organic local food systems.

While the movement's cultural roots extend to ancient Greece, the official inauguration of the Slow Philosophy took place in Italy. In 1989, Carlo Petrini, then a freelance restaurant reviewer with a genius for politics, staged a protest against the new McDonald's in Rome's fabled Piazza di Spagna. The protesters made their point by sitting outside the fast food multinational, very slowly eating bowls of homemade pasta.

This delectable – and globally reported – rebellion had been building for years. Three years earlier, Arcigola, a Piedmont-based group dedicated to the education of local food producers and what Petrini, now sixty-five, called "awakening people's attention to wine and food and the right way to enjoy them", had organized its first tasting courses. In December 1989, Petrini and delegates from fourteen countries met in Paris to establish the first Slow Food manifesto and authorize the movement's logo: a snail. The Slow Food manifesto was entitled, "International Movement in Defense of the Right to Pleasure".

Slow Food, a nonprofit organization, now employs over 100 people and involves millions of people in 150 countries. Its impact on our eating habits has been inestimable. Since the mid-1990s, it has been government accredited to train teachers about food and eating, and in 2004 it founded the University of Gastronomic Sciences. Slow Food also established the Ark of Taste to prevent seeds, raw foodstuffs and culinary traditions from being made extinct, and it now endorses sustainable agriculture. The core belief is simple: that "everyone has a fundamental right to the pleasure of good food and consequently the responsibility to protect the heritage of biodiversity, culture and knowledge that make this pleasure possible".

Petrini, who, as the organization's founder and president, is on first name terms with Barack Obama, Al Gore, David Cameron and Prince Charles (who calls him "My dear Carlo"), has always associated food with pleasure. "My memories of food are of the dishes my grandmother used to prepare", he recalls. "This was the culinary tradition of Piedmont, the region of Northern Italy where I was born and live. The Piedmontese tradition is based on simple ingredients, very tasty, and varied. This area at the foot of the Alps was once quite poor, so many traditional dishes, such as finanziera, are made using all parts of animals, or the ravioli were filled with meat leftovers and rice and cabbage."

The elegant and surprisingly slender Petrini believes that pleasure in dining is fundamental to a happy life and that such pleasure can only be restored through the culture of food, or "eco-gastronomy", as he calls it. "Culture is essential", he explains. "There can be no pleasure without knowledge, and no knowledge without pleasure. If people know more about food they will enjoy it more, feel more involved."

Thinking about what to eat and food preparation are some of life's deepest pleasures, he maintains. He deplores celebrity chefs. Their programs, he believes, are "pornography", and nothing like the "act of love" that is cooking for those we love.

"Dining, then, can be an important convivial moment with family and friends", he says. "Sitting at a table together, enjoying good food, having the opportunity for conversation. If food is genuine, it is a pleasure, makes us feel good, and doesn't pollute the body with chemical additives. Food isn't just fuel, but something that holds the utmost importance as it becomes part of the physical self; we literally are what we eat."

Petrini's words and actions have caused thousands to stop and register – perhaps for the first time – how devoid of deep pleasure their lives have come to feel.

Carl Honoré, forty-eight, whose international bestseller *In Praise of Slow* transformed the peripatetic Scottish–Canadian newspaper stringer into the mouthpiece for the Slow Movement, in part blames the IT revolution for the lowering of our quality of life.

"We now put a premium on high speed and instant delivery, with everything reduced to a 140-character tweet", he says. "As speed occupies more of a cultural space, less of a cultural space has been allocated to contemplation, which belongs to the slower track. And the more activities are marginalized, the more they come to be seen as a crime or offensive. We're on a trend, here. Men are particularly vulnerable as there is a kind of machismo attached to speed. We reward the fastest and that taps into competition."

Norwegian physicist and psychologist Geir Berthelsen, fifty, agrees. In 1999, Berthelsen founded the World Institute of Slowness, a Slow Revolution think tank. His favourite challenges are those pertaining to change management, stress, creativity, problem solving and process improvements in what he calls our "firefighting" culture.

"The fast will beat the big, but the Slow will beat the fast", he maintains.

The jolly Berthelsen notes that our culture's omnipresent corporate mindset is "long on quantity and short on quality. The focus is on the end product, not on the process itself. In the West, the man with the most toys wins, and not the man with the most time to play with the toys. Ironically, the best business thinking often comes from a walk in the Slow lane. We have forgotten that there is more than one dimension to time. We have something to learn from the ancient Greeks, who believed that time has two dimensions: Chronos and Kairos. Chronos being linear time and Kairos being the time when special events happen, what the Greeks called 'the supreme moment'."

Time, Honoré concurs, is the new currency. In the West, he says, "time is linear, an arrow flying remorselessly from A to B – a finite, and therefore precious, resource".

Ironically, Honoré, whose charming, erudite and intense demeanour is that of the hero of a 1940s newsroom film noir, loves speed. He relishes deadlines, a fast internet connection, ice-hockey and squash, and lives in London, "a city of volcanic energy". "I've always had a fast natural pace, so in some ways I was easy prey for the cult of speed", he laughs. "The virus of hurry found it easy to get into my bloodstream!"

His second bestseller, *Under Pressure: How the Epidemic of Hyper-Parenting is Endangering Childhood*, was, aptly, written under pressure: how to follow a book that sold over half a million copies in thirty languages? "I was stunned when *In Praise of Slow* became a hit", he admits. "As it was coming out, I was already making plans to return to journalism. The book not only seemed to touch a nerve, but just keeps gaining momentum. I think it has become a kind of touchstone, part of the cultural furniture. The gratifying aspect was that it has been used as a tool for changing things for the better."

Honoré remembers summers as feeling very slow in childhood, and having a sense of time as being expansive: days and days and days stretched out ahead of him. His family home had a large backyard and trees into which he would disappear for hours on end. "I clearly remember swinging on the cherry tree when it was in full blossom", he says, "thinking that I could just swing there forever, just … lightness".

Such moments are much more than pleasing, he believes; they are priceless. "Those are the moments that help to define your childhood, the memory of who you were, and the foundation of your identity", he explains. "That open-ended, untrammelled, free play is what small children do to knock their brains into shape; there are developmental reasons behind wafting around a tree all day, inventing games and weaving narratives around the ladybirds you find on leaves. But there is also a glorious romantic magic about it – the soaring, simple joy of being a child. That world William Blake wrote about:

To see a world in a grain of sand,
And a heaven in a wild flower,
Hold infinity in the palm of your hand,
And eternity in an hour.

That sense of possibility, adventure, freedom."

Honoré remembers that the slowness, that sense of infinite excitement, possibility and adventure, disappeared when he started working in journalism. He began to feel as if he were racing through his life rather than actually living it. "Speed delivers a superficial experience of the world", he says. "I was just ticking boxes. I didn't feel like I was present or fully connected with anything or anyone. I couldn't be in the moment, because I was often in several moments at once, or worse; I was worrying about the next moment, or the moment after that, or trying to juggle two moments at the same time. And that's the way the whole culture was moving – everybody was online all the time, mobiles on 24/7, Blackberrys: all this was happening in parallel to my own roadrunner existence."

Speed, Honoré says, is like a drug, and our civilization is addicted. Other than the adrenaline rush, speed also has a metaphysical dimension. Individually and collectively, it serves as a mechanism of denial, a means of avoiding the bigger questions. "If you're rushing around", he explains, "you don't have time to ask yourself who you really are, what your purpose is, or whether you're leaving the world a better place. Because all you have time to ask is: Where have I put my keys? I'm late for my 11am! People sense something's wrong, but instead of slowing down to deal with it, they go even faster and eventually slam into a brick wall. People say, 'My wakeup call came when I couldn't get out of bed one day'. Or, 'My back seized up'. Often, the body revolts; it's had enough."

Idler co-founder Hodgkinson, whose first book, *How to Be Idle*, is published in twenty countries, has an entirely less charitable view of the system. "Look", he says as he sips a cup of tea, "I think the whole Slow Movement is really good – I even subscribe to the Slow Food magazine. However, I'm a little more politically radical. Slow Living tells you to slow down and de-stress within the corporation – you know, Slow human resources counsellors telling employers to do things more slowly in order to have more happier and therefore more productive employees, bigger profits and no strikes. But I'm not about being happy in the system; I'm about finding new ways to be happy."

Hodgkinson is not at all a layabout but a flâneur, at once an anarchist and epicurean. To this end, he works "very hard" from 9am to 1pm every day. Sometimes he even unplugs the phone and the internet. He then has a short nap, prepares the house for the return of his three young children from school, and, in the evening, is his wife's sous-chef: chopping vegetables, preparing drinks. When not strumming the ukulele – the cover of the bestselling *How to Be Free* has him sitting on a grocery cart, strumming – he does an "enormous" amount of housework. (But if he is playing the ukulele in the kitchen and his wife walks in, he quietly puts it down and carries on with the washing up.)

"I never stop!" he squeaks, sounding unnervingly like Hugh Grant. "I'm always cleaning and washing up. I do all the gardening, vegetable-growing and poultry-keeping. And I do the wood-chopping and storage and lighting the fires, all big jobs. We have had cleaners, but we can't afford it anymore. It never really worked anyway, because they'd clean for three hours, leave, and then five minutes later, the house was a shit-hole again."

In his most recent book, *The Idle Parent*, he argues, like Honoré, that childhood is being sacrificed to the gross national product. Over-scheduling and parental work-related absences are encouraged, he says, because they boost the economy. "Just sitting around at home – not working, not spending money – doesn't actually contribute to economic growth, which is why idleness is not advertised particularly widely", he says, shaking his head. "Western women are encouraged to go back to work very quickly after having a baby. Separation is key. Must encourage separation! I've looked into the history of the Protestant work ethic, and in the Protestant theology, people are actually separated from each other and from God. So in our culture, you're supposed to be a separated, isolated individual on a lonely course through life, that dismal pilgrimage."

Hodgkinson comes from a family of high-profile journalists. His mother, Liz, and father, Neville, were boldface Fleet Street regulars, and his brother, Will, is a renowned music journalist. They have written over sixty books between them. "Which just shows how unimaginative we are", Hodgkinson sighs. "My mother always used to make money writing about us when we were little boys, so now we do the same about them. It's called revenge. My mother's pieces were never particularly positive, you see. She once wrote that she would rather clean the kitchen floor than play with us. Our lives were exploited."

In Hodgkinson's teens, his parents "went quite weird". Between the ages of thirteen to nineteen, he had a "house full of Indian ladies wearing dhotis because my father got into meditation. He's still into it. He loved being celibate, which was a bonus for my mother, I think. She went along with the meditation thing so far, got fed up with it, and they split." He pauses. "My brother and I both turned out reasonably well, although my wife would disagree, but I think I'm reasonably not mentally ill – given my background, I mean."

Hodgkinson, forever damned as lazy, made heroes of historical loafers, if only to make himself feel better. Samuel Johnson, "a great loafer", may have written the first English language dictionary, but he was also, it seems, a great idler. "John Lennon was also extremely lazy. He wrote lots of songs in praise of loafing around, watching the wheels turn, and so on. Oscar Wilde, too, enjoyed discussion of idleness as an activity". Cultivated leisure as a noble pursuit is, he concedes, an aristocratic ideal. "Well, yes", he says, embarrassed. "It comes from the Greeks and the Romans, who had slaves. The free man had the liberty to cultivate his leisure and indulge in the arts and rhetoric and philosophy. Such pursuits are characteristic of the free man, not the slave."

Where Hodgkinson differs from the aristocracy is this: he believes in shouldering, rather than delegating, the care of one's own children. "That's a reality of today", he says. "We don't have slaves, we *are* slaves. It's just not possible today to have a household of servants. Sometimes I wish it were. I read about the Edwardian writers – they had all these cooks and maids and butlers. They must have had so much time to write. They didn't have to do the washing up and the cleaning and the cooking." He pauses. "Seriously, though: my idea of idleness does not depend on the toil of others."

Hodgkinson mostly blames television for our widespread commodification. "Years ago, I bought a very large TV", he remembers. "I'd come down at five-thirty in the morning with my eldest and watch television for two or three hours. The effects were obvious. He became unable to entertain himself. The world jumps in early these days. TV's all over hospitals now – in maternity wards, everywhere. You're commodified the moment you're born. You must spend money! And that's what TV's all about. Unplugging the box, though, is surprisingly difficult. People think you're insane, but it's essential for sanity. These days, people watch cooking programmes instead of cooking, gardening programmes instead of gardening, and porn instead of making love. Madness."

Frequently photographed dishevelled on an unkempt lawn as their pre-Raphaelite children whirl about them, Hodgkinson and his wife enjoy Slow Love, an increasingly rare state of intimacy in the West. Despite being together all day for close to a decade, Hodgkinson still mentions his wife every few minutes, and with the kind of exasperated affection known only to the uxorious.

"We do feel lucky", he says, and then retracts the comment, claiming he doesn't want to seem like one of Bridget Jones' "Smug Marrieds".

He exhales. "Look, it's very, very hard on a marriage when the children are small – it's kind of a nightmare, actually. I've loads of friends who are divorcing; in some cases, perhaps they were too idle. We've been through really difficult periods – tired, grouchy, arguing over small things, both feeling overstretched and that the other person is not doing enough, or doing it wrong. But then I remember that at the beginning of the financial collapse, bankers had bottles thrown at their heads by their wives, who were screaming LOSER! at them because they were no longer able to support the staff."

Nurturing the soul, Hodgkinson says, is critical, "because otherwise, you always have a slight, nagging anxiety that something's wrong. That's how I used to feel all the time when I worked in London." His yelp is sudden. "Oh my God, I've gotta go – Victoria is going to kill me if I don't take those potatoes out of the oven!"

Slow Love makes for significantly greater intimacy between

couples and, in sexual matters, deeper pleasure. Similarly, Slow Sex acolytes emphasise communication and tenderness above impersonal, masturbatory sex, explaining that at core, all people desire to love and to be loved and that love – or love-making – simply cannot be forced. As our expectations of self have become more mechanistic, our relationships have become less fulfilling: reduced to function, stripped of romance and, increasingly, shallow.

"It's even welded into the vernacular of human resources," Honoré exclaims. "People are now regarded as no more than assets on the balance sheet. We've sped everything else up, so why not speed up human relations? But you can't make someone fall in love with you in May because you want to get married in June. You can't forge a friendship more quickly because you need a backpacking companion around Europe. Relationships have a natural, universal, timeless rhythm. So you have with this absurd situation where you have 921 friends on Facebook, but when was the last time you spent an afternoon in the park chatting to any of them? We end up with quantity over quality."

Civility, by definition, is dependent on slowness, if only because the needs of others have to be taken into consideration. The small respectful courtesies that make everyday life pleasurable are sacrificed in the rush to get on to the next thing.

"More and more, people approach others as if they were props", Honoré says. "That's why a tsunami of pornography has washed over our culture. Porn is the ultimate commodification of the ultimate act of intimacy; it is the apex of sexual efficiency. The thing about romance is that it's slow – in the making, in the enjoyment, in the remembering. The antithesis of romance is efficiency. When things speed up, one of the first casualties is romance, which is why our culture is so uncomfortable with romance – all kinds, not just in matters of love. The romance of art, of pleasure, of thought … we don't have the time! We gotta get the experience under our belts and onto our CVs."

Life without romance, he observes, is a very flat, grey thing. "Romance ennobles and animates us and is at the core of being alive, whether it's the romance of passion or life itself. I think we've created a culture that is so driven by management principles that we've become obsessed with outcomes. We have lost the art of the journey, and that's where romance resides. Doing things for the sake of doing them."

Honoré has observed that our culture is predicated on the ideas that faster is better and more is more. "Which is why you make yourself more attractive, more efficient and more modern by accelerating – doing more and more with less and less time", he says. "That's hardwired into the DNA of the twenty-first century. The whole consumer industry is pushing us to spend, spend, spend. You see people on trains, planes, buses – they never sit there any more and just think; they're always fiddling with their phones or iPhones or iPods. People feel that if they're disconnected for even fifteen minutes, their stock will fall."

He pauses. "But the tectonic plates are shifting. More and more people are waking up to the fact that faster isn't always better. It has become obvious to many that we need to rethink our approaches to time, life and the way we run the world."

Pretor-Pinney is regularly asked by his fellow cloud enthusiasts if he can join them for a spot of cloudspotting, but, as he explains, "it doesn't really work like that. And that's the beauty of it: not planning. Clouds don't do what you want them to do. You have to be receptive and stop what you're doing when you notice something."

Somerset, the Pretor-Pinney family's new home, has "lots of perfect spots for cloudspotting because there are so few obstructions to the sky". Their house is a converted barn – it was once the cowshed next to his parents' house – situated on a little lane that ends in the woods. "Probably half the village was conceived in that barn", he giggles. His favourite room is his office, which is lined with books and has a little wood-burning stove.

He believes it essential for men to learn to live slowly, if only to recover the sense of joy and liberty in being. "By slowing down, by finding the beauty in the everyday, the mundane, you learn to focus on the journey rather than the destination. That said, it can be difficult. I feel torn between the two ways of looking at the world, too; but the Cloud Appreciation Society, *The Cloudspotter's Guide* and *The Wavewatcher's Companion* are all successful examples of having no goals at all – all three started as casual ideas and evolved organically. I never want to retire, you see. Retirement is the secular afterlife; you work hard at some crappy job and then retire to play golf. Whereas I want to have learned the secret of incorporating my work and life so that the pleasure is in both – I want to reach the state where I can't remember whether I'm working or playing."

Geir Berthelsen's ten-point guide to going slow

1. Set your alarm clock always ten minutes before you need to get up. (You will never run late.)
2. Prepare and eat a structured breakfast – for example, from 06:45 – 07:10 every day.
3. Let all involved parties – children and parents – talk during the breakfast and say what they think the highlight of the coming day will be. LISTEN.
4. Hug each other before leaving the house.
5. Smile. Try it!
6. Don't skip lunch.
7. At 2 pm each day, ask yourself: "How am I feeling?"
8. Prepare and eat dinner with the whole family – no television on – and let everyone recount the highlights of their day. LISTEN.
9. Exercise for at least 20 minutes per day. Take a short walk, even if it's raining.
10. Before bed, spend five minutes reviewing the day and plan tomorrow's highlights.

Don't live life as if you are afraid of being late to your own funeral!

worldinstituteofslowness.com

One from the heart

A conversation with Steve Biddulph

What you have to do is surrender to life and allow yourself to be helpless, and out of that, if you stay with it, comes the liberation.

Anglo-Australian psychologist Steve Biddulph may be a gentle man, as courteous to the wombats he rehabilitates as he is to the families he counsels, but his challenge to the corporatization of human beings is uncompromising. His aim is true: to return us to our hearts. Biddulph's simply written books, now translated into twenty-seven languages, have sold in the millions, and include *Raising Boys: Why Boys Are Different – and How to Help Them Become Happy and Well-Balanced Men*; *The Secret of Happy Children: Why Children Behave the Way They Do – and What You Can Do to Help Them to be Optimistic*; *Manhood*; and *Raising Babies*. Despite this, he is resolutely opposed to the branding that characterizes certain other childcare experts. There is no capped smile, no Botox, no contacts, and he is unremittingly awkward. "I think it's fairly likely that I have mild Asperger's", he notes. Comfortingly human, he both appeals to and elicits the very best in people. Voted Australian Father of the Year in 2000 for his efforts to increase the involvement of fathers with their children, the sixty-one-year-old Biddulph is outspoken about both the institutionalization of infants and the premature sexualization of children. "There is no poetry left", he has said. "For the boys, conditioned by online porn and compliant but disengaged girls, sex may come to have no more meaning than an ice cream or a pizza. For millions of girls, sex has become a performance, anxiously overlaid with worry about how do I look? What sexual tricks does he expect or not expect? How do I compare with all the others he has slept with? Little wonder we have one of the most depressed, anxious and lonely generations of young people ever." Now based in Tasmania, he and Shaaron, his wife of four decades and the mother of his two children, fund projects for the betterment of the community, notably the Sanctuary Refugee Trust and the SIEV X memorial.

AGB: I remember taking Bethesda into the CBD for lunch with some girlfriends. She was three years old at the time. And as I walked through the city with her, two men came close to hitting her in the face with their briefcases; they were so preoccupied, they didn't even bother to look where they were going. The only people who engaged with her in any way – the only people who noticed that there was a little child in their midst – were of Asian or European background. I was astounded.

SB: The cultural capacity for love can be lost. In America, upper-class women specify that the carers who apply to look after their children are Hispanic –

AGB: In certain elite New York hospitals, they actually provide interpreters so the Hispanic nannies can take over the minute the baby is born.

SB: We are outsourcing love to the developing world. And women wonder why their husbands fall in love with the nanny!

AGB: Jude Law, Arnold Schwarzenegger, the late Robin Williams and Ethan Hawke all did it, which is why Victoria Beckham's nannies do not look like Scarlett Johansson. Aristocratic women throughout the centuries have always delegated mothering, which is, in part, why women are encouraged to delegate mothering today. It's part of the aspirational package.

SB: The affluent are the biggest users of childcare, absolutely.

AGB: Is that right?

SB: Parents can be divided into three groups: those who don't use child care at all, those who slide into childcare gradually as the kiddies get to two or three years of age, and what we call the slammers. The slammers parent one in twenty children. By and large, slammers are overwhelmingly affluent, two-career-centred parents. So the delegation isn't driven by financial need. Although you do get a sort of collateral effect – house prices mainly rise on the phenomenon of the two-income family, who can bid for a higher price, and so the housing market has climbed. And what this means is that a lot of other people have been forced to have two incomes. But blue-collar people, and especially blue-collar immigrants, will resist using stranger care as much as they possibly can.

AGB: The issue is an incendiary one. There were calls to ban author Mem Fox's books when she reported that a childcare worker had told her: "We're going to look back on this time from the late nineties onward – with putting children in child-care so early in their first year of life for such long hours – and wonder how we have allowed that child abuse to happen."

SB: Seventy per cent of parents here feel that children under three shouldn't go to daycare. Because if you haven't ever had this kind of nurturing, you literally don't know what it's about. It's like women who had absent or mostly absent fathers – they see no value in having husbands or fathers for their children. It's deeply unconscious stuff that repeats through the generations. Aristocratic families, for thousands of years, didn't know how to love their children.

AGB: A dear friend – an erudite, deep-feeling, brilliant man, was enrolled in boarding school at the age of four. Four! At the age of fifty, he finally mustered the courage to ask his mother why she had done this to him, and she replied, "It was very hard". And that was the end of the conversation.

SB: Prince Charles is a classic example. His mother went on a six-month tour when he was four; he stayed in England. There's footage of him meeting the royal aircraft on its return. The Queen came down the steps of the plane and this little boy with an overcoat on shook her hand!

AGB: His adored nanny, Mimsy, looked exactly like –

SB: Camilla Parker Bowles?

AGB: Yes! They could be twins.

SB: An infant doesn't give a damn whether it's born under a hedge or in a tin shack or a palace; the location doesn't even register. But newborns are acutely aware of their mother's happiness. And so the emotional environment around birth is of paramount importance. A little baby will scan the pupils of your eyes every sixty seconds or so, and they can tell if you're feeling relaxed and attentive because your pupils will be dilated. If your pupils contract, they start to get nervy. A baby's stress levels rise and fall with its mother's. There's even a study of premature babies showing that if their parents look down into the humidicrib, the premmie will monitor the relationship between the mother and the father. The mechanism isn't properly understood. It's as if the baby needs to know that mum is safe, and that dad loves mum. And if that's the case, the baby rocks into a safe state, and when they're in that state, their growth hormones increase. So growth hormones enter the brain and the parts of the brain that govern paying attention, being calm and feeling focused develop more quickly. We now think that ADHD is caused in the second six months of life –

AGB: When the ability to bond is forged? Really?

SB: Yes! And if you have a mother who's extremely stressed in the second six months of life, then she won't be able to provide the focus that the child needs to develop that part of the cortex. ADHD needs a genetic predisposition as a certain amount of it is inherited, but if you have the predisposition and a calm mother, it won't develop; if, on the other hand, you have the predisposition and a stressed mother, then the disorder is likely to manifest. The occipital frontal cortex is measurably thinner in people with ADHD, and so it's looking like the interaction between babies and their primary caretakers are of crucial importance, particularly in the second six months. That's when babies get really fussy about their caretakers. The second six months of life is when the really fine stuff happens – by that stage, the mother knows the baby's signals so well. Researchers have filmed the interactions between mothers and babies using the sorts of cameras that stop bullets, and there are exchanges between mother and child where they cannot separate who started it.

AGB: Complete synchronicity.

SB: It's through the fineness of the interaction with the mother that babies learn this sensing of people so they can get their timing right in adulthood, because intimacy is basically a timing thing.

AGB: Sensitivity to others is one of the greatest gifts we can give our children.

SB: Exactly. The biggest concern in the mental health field is that it is possible to simply not learn intimacy. You get these human beings who often have very good superficial people skills – and this comes out of the child-care thing: they're very slick, very charming, or whatever's needed to get the results, but there's no connection behind it. And then you get marriages where it's really more of an economic team situation than anything else. There's an epidemic of an inability to be close.

AGB: What sort of intimacy issues are suffered by children deprived of their mothers?

SB: It's mothers that you learn intimacy from. The first six years of life are about learning to be close, and usually that's mum at the centre and then dad and hopefully two or three other people – aunts and uncles, grandparents. Emotional literacy is the foundation of intelligence. And yet we see it the other way around – you're intelligent and maybe have some emotional intelligence on the side to give you some people skills. In fact, the way the brain is put together, the emotions are there and everything else is built on top of that. All this rubbish with *Baby Einstein* DVDs and things actually interrupts that. Studies show that children shouldn't be around screens for the first three years or so at all because then they don't get the proper visual clues.

AGB: It has reached the point where the lack of intimacy has been normalized. Those who seek intimacy are regarded either as zealots or as enemies of the corporate state.

SB: Mass nursery care was introduced around Dickens' time. The reforming people of Lady Gowrie's era figured that since babies were being cared for in horrible circumstances, anything they could do to improve that had to be a plus. Hygienic-trained, responsible daycare was a revolution of the 1950s. Its usage quadrupled in the 1980s or thereabouts, especially with very, very little babies.

AGB: How does this tie into our capacity to love?

SB: The negative parenting that was happening in the 1970s and 1980s was the biggest issue; that's when we really started losing the capacity to love. Are you familiar with the Indian concept of a juggernaut? It's a huge cart that is wheeled through the town, and actually crushes people to death as it goes through because it's so huge; the only way people can steer it is by throwing themselves at it en masse to push or jolt it around the corner. And I see Western culture the same way.

AGB: So you see yourself as helping steer the juggernaut?

SB: I do.

AGB: Explain to me how we understand the concept of family in this culture.

SB: That's where we have a problem. A family would normally be thirty or forty people connected by blood, and that's how we lived for 300,000 years. Every single piece of our wiring is geared to that. We even have slots in our brains for uncles and aunties, who come in and balance the perfectly normal deficiencies of mum and dad. We were made to live in that matrix. The two-parent family we have today is a fragment, and it won't work. This is probably the main message of twenty-first century psychology. A nuclear family can only get a child to twelve; from twelve onward, the child will become dysfunctional unless there's another circle of adults around the family. So you have to build tribal connections early on. You've got to have people who love your children from when they're so high, so by the time they're teenagers, those people are available to them. If you can, don't relocate, don't lose friendships, don't neglect people. Invest in friends, because they'll be the difference between life and death to you when your children are teenagers. The day will come when you can't stand your own children, and vice versa – they'll storm out of the house, go round the corner to your friend's house, spend the night there, and cry about how terrible you are, and your friend's kids come the opposite way, doing the same – sometimes they pass in the street!

AGB: Forty supportive relatives? My husband and I have four.

SB: I often have conversations about this with people, and tell them what they need to do, and they say, "But implementing those changes would be difficult!" As if everything's supposed to be easy. It's not, you know? This is something that ought to be written in the sky: life is really, really, really hard. Yes, it's joyful and fantastic, but it will also tear you in half any number of times. And the two hardest things are parenthood and staying married. The idea that there's a fix or a book or a workshop or some guru who will say, "Here, just do this and life will be easy!", is ridiculous.

AGB: I've observed a chasm between societal expectations of women these days and motherhood. Fundamental human needs are clashing with status-based desires.

SB: There have been a lot of colliding ideologies. Feminism told women that they'd submerged themselves in the needs of others and had to address their own needs – which was really important, because it was true. Mothers literally did not have a self in the old family model. But then it went overboard. One of the things that parenthood involves is this really big shift from coming first to coming second to this little creature in your life. The brains of committed parents actually change. When you're available to your baby around the clock, everything changes. Prolactin floods into your bloodstream from breastfeeding, and even the father's brain changes.

AGB: You wrote very movingly in *Raising Babies* about daycare from the child's perspective; I was in tears. Why have we been conditioned to understand wanting attention as a weakness?

SB: Again, it's a splitting-off from the heart. People deal with a difficult childhood by splitting off from their hearts; it's a survival skill. If somebody sends out heart-messages through need, it activates your own heart, and if you've deadened your heart, you deal with them the way you deal with yourself. The same coldness that was shown to you, you will use toward yourself. And you will use that coldness with those who give off the same signals of need. So it's a struggle. It's the same reason people rape and beat children. Everything that's done to a child, they will do to others.

AGB: So how do we stop this toxic cycle?

SB: We need to find the circuit-breaker. The answer is finding the heart-connection. As a therapist, what I say to a family having troubles is – let's say it's between father and daughter or mother and daughter – go away together for forty-eight hours. Go up the coast, go anywhere. Because you shouldn't always go everywhere as a family. Say dad and daughter go away for a couple of days. What they'll have is a showdown, the catch-up fight that's been waiting to happen. But if the dad knows that's on the cards, he'll stay grounded and he'll hear what his teenage daughter has to say; he'll weather it out. Through the cycle of being together, of cooking and sleeping and going through the cycle of day and night, they'll have the opportunity to make a heart-connection.

AGB: My father once tried that with me. We flew to Europe; the idea was to drive from Northern Italy through to Paris. We lasted five days.

SB: Too ambitious. There's a trade secret of family therapy, called the 5-per-cent rule. A 5-per-cent change in a system is a sustainable change. If you were to change a family by 10 per cent, they'd go into shock because there would be just too much shaking up. We were taught to aim for a 5-per-cent change because a year later, another 5-per-cent can be effected.

AGB: So you're not an advocate of emotional shock therapy?

SB: Very, very rarely. If you want to help other people to change, it has to be in increments.

AGB: One thing I've noticed is a significant decrease in emotional literacy. I mean, there is a world of difference between the people I meet in the course of my everyday life and, say, my great-uncle, whose emotional literacy was extraordinary. He read people the way I would read a book. It was such a pleasure to be with him, such a pleasure to feel known.

SB: Shakespeare's audiences were street apprentices. The aristocrats went to see his plays as well, but most of the people in his audience flowed in from the streets. People were vastly more articulate and nuanced in interpersonal communication. The level of language alone! Same with Dickens.

AGB: There has been a marked degradation in both emotional literacy and literacy in general since the advent of television.

SB: Television has dumbed us down.

AGB: What would happen, do you think, if people disconnected their sets? Would that be a 5-per-cent change?

SB: [laughing] That would be a 100-per-cent change! TV's huge! It structures your time and does all sorts of things. One of my interests is in hunter-gatherer cultures, because they had much smarter kids and much better sensory development. We've lived in trashed cultures for 200 years.

AGB: Do you think the parents of young children should bin their television sets?

SB: Yes. But I go for achievable goals. First, never have a television in a child's bedroom. We know that this effects a huge improvement in the child's mental health. Second, watch designated programs. Don't have a TV running all the time.

AGB: Why?

SB: There's this thing with play. A toddler will verbalize to themselves continuously as they play, and they're probably doing amazing things for their language while they're doing it. But if you have a television or a radio on in the background, it eliminates 80 per cent of the child's verbalizing. It blocks the channels. So the child is blocked by the daytime soaps or whatever's on the news, because they haven't learned to filter noise out yet. If the TV's on, the child won't do that play. Instead, it will become listless and just aimlessly wander about. We really have to look at the auditory environment we put our children in. Just leave the environment alone, you know? Leave it unpolluted so the child can fill out. The Steiner people make dolls without any features, and it's really sophisticated thinking as the child projects onto the blank face.

AGB: Bethesda used to play families with a set of spoons! She used to say, "This is the mama spoon, and this is the dadda spoon, and you have to give me another spoon so I can make a little baby." How do you feel about children only being permitted to have computers in family spaces?

SB: The general thinking is yes, children should only access the internet in family spaces because of what's on the net. Children should never access computers in private spaces because if they do, at some point they'll come across pornography and they'll get engaged.

AGB: I've read so many uninformed comments about parental responsibility – you know, "It's up to parents to police their children; the rest of us should be able to access anything we want". As if it's possible to police children 24/7. That would involve grilling the parents, relatives and older siblings of your child's friends – in addition to all their friends – and inspecting all their iPhones and PCs. I mean, how do we protect our children from pornography? How do you arm a six-year-old who is shown pornographic material by a friend's older sibling?

SB: I was talking to a man whose six-year-old son made a little friend over the road. The boy asked his father if he could go over to his new friend's house to play; the father said yes. When the man went to pick his son up at tea time, there was hardcore porn on the coffee table. So he had to explain his son that he was no longer allowed to go to his friend's house and that it was really sad, but there was no other solution.

AGB: What do you say to a child who has been exposed to pornography?

SB: You find out what their concerns are, listen to their questions, and deal with those. I will never forget the day my son asked from his car seat, "Why did they kill that baby?" Shaaron and I pulled over. We didn't make a big drama, but asked, "Did we hear right?" Turns out he'd heard about the murder on a news broadcast the day before. He'd sat on it for twenty-four hours before speaking about it. Back then, we thought that kids didn't really pay attention to that sort of thing, but after that there was no more news at our place! I mean, imagine what kids are doing with reports of rape and murder and porn and so on.

AGB: It's just so sad. What are the effects of this kind of material on infant and toddler brains?

SB: Again, they'll do that splitting thing, where they think, "I won't feel that". They'll have to invest a certain amount of psychic energy in not feeling whatever it is they're too frightened to feel, and during the process, they'll become more and more removed from themselves. In therapy, when you see someone in recovery or getting through something, there will be layers and layers of stuff that they thought didn't trouble them at the time, and when one layer's removed, then the next one comes to the surface. Jean Liedloff's book, *The Continuum Concept*, was amazing. In it, she recorded her travels with tribespeople of the Amazon. The Indians had a fair bit of medical gear, so they could do medical procedures. She watched as this big, tough Amazon man put his head on his wife's lap, sobbing, as he stuck his thumb out to be amputated – without an anaesthetic – and when it was done, he'd be fine, because he'd discharged his feelings in a totally normal way. They would feel a feeling and then let it go. There was no residue, no complication.

AGB: Liedloff said that we oppose our babies from the start, allowing ourselves to be led by society rather than by our own feelings. "We wage a war of wills", she wrote. The baby is sobbing with hunger and we say, "No, it's not time for you to eat!" Wouldn't it be extraordinary to live in a culture that allowed human beings emotional breadth?

SB: Children are great, because they naturally express their feelings. Whenever comfort's available, they'll discharge whatever tension they've accumulated. Have you heard of co-counselling?

AGB: I haven't, no.

SB: You meet weekly with a co-counsellor and give each other half an hour of undivided attention to release the stress you've built up in the course of the week. It's very freeing. Because most people in urban environments are basket cases.

AGB: The noise levels alone – traffic, aircraft, TV, radio and so on – are so anxiety-making.

SB: As a culture, we're losing headspace. We need to put rhythm back in childhood. People are gradually realizing this. A kid gets more out of one fully digested experience than twenty experiences at partial attention.

AGB: When Bethesda was so tiny that she couldn't even roll over, I made her aware of her face by gently tracing a finger over every part of it – her little nose, her septum, her brow. Her expressions were so beautiful. Now, you've written that the most significant factor of all in determining child mental health is maternal sensitivity. If a mother is low on sensitivity, how can she improve?

SB: I've never thought of that. Wow. I think it's the enlivening you were talking about before the interview – incorporating passion into your life – and slowing down, really. It's probably a personal bias, but having a spiritual dimension to your life – either meditating or praying or doing yoga or going to church or temple, anything. The spiritual dimension is beyond talk. It's starting to let your boundaries dissolve and being more connected to life. We really need to remove a lot of the stresses around mothers so they can have more transitional experiences. Mothers need to do anything they can do to slow themselves, to calm themselves. I would say this to any mother who has issues with sensitivity: You are intrinsically designed to be a responsive mother; it's in you to do that. Your hormones are primed to flow; you just need to get out of your own way. People talk about spirituality, but it's just surrendering. There's a river of life running through you. If you picture a line of human history, all 300,000 years of it, it would be a line of mothers going back for fifty miles. And in a sense, it's actually there. Because the caring of all those mothers was effective enough for you to be here. You can literally lean back into that. So if you're conscious of what's actually on your side and working for you, then ego doesn't even come into it. You were made for this.

AGB: How can we restore value to the idea of family?

SB: The commodity that we're most short of is time. There are places in the world where the issue is food or safety, but with us it's time. So if you increase the amount of time between any two human beings, the amount of love will start to grow. Because it's just a natural consequence of people being together in the same space. If you're concerned about a relationship, just feed it with time. It won't be instant bliss; the friction and the irritation and the baggage will come to the fore, and if that's digested and given its chance to play out, good things will happen. Because intimacy is about friction as well as connection. You need to work out your priorities, which most people don't stop to do. What actually makes people happy is helping others. We're here for each other. Life only makes sense if you look at the big picture. People are miserable until they begin to serve.

AGB: But you can only be of service when you've sorted yourself out. A car that doesn't work shouldn't be used to transport others.

SB: Where I think you're wrong is that you never have yourself sorted out.

AGB: I disagree. There's a baseline of functionality.

SB: People should just start being of service, then they can work on each other.

AGB: Ted Bundy worked for a suicide hotline, but I don't think it did him much good! [laughs] You've addressed the urge for independence as a mask for fear in mothers – underneath the feeling of being burdened, you wrote, is the fear that they're inadequate or can't meet the child's needs.

SB: I remember reading an article where a fashion model said that she stayed home with her baby for six months, but then she "needed her independence". What she really meant was that she needed her freedom. Not to have the burden of a human being there. But independence sounded more edifying. Independence is often behind a fear of closeness. There's a thing that happens with mothers and little babies. It can be shattering to realise that you will never have a full night's sleep again and that for the foreseeable future, you won't be able to do anything when you want to do it. For a lot of people, that's so, so shocking. Or for a professional woman, who's always been so organized and effective, to realise that she just can't stop this baby crying.

AGB: A complete overhaul of self-image.

SB: What you have to do is surrender to life and allow yourself to be helpless, and out of that, if you stay with it, comes the liberation. But if you back off and run away, it won't happen for you. It's much like having a disabled baby. The first response, particularly of the husband is: "I don't wanna know! Put it in an institution! Let's get out of here and start again! Don't even think about it!" The next point is, "All right, what do I do? How can I help?" Which then evolves into, "I love this child, and I'm so glad I have this child in my life." All of those stages have to be lived, and if you deny the despair, you'll never have the liberation. So you have to go down into the trough to come out. The redemptive suffering leads to equanimity. We all need to fall to bits every six months; we all need to regularly come unstuck. Because if you tough it out, put on more make-up, a braver face, you'll just crash further down the track. What's needed in this culture is people who encourage parents to experience the grief and loss of what they thought their lives were about.

AGB: So interesting. The same is true of so many relationships. People just don't stick it out. I'm not talking about dangerous or deadening situations, but rocky periods. And the culture supports this; we're encouraged to walk, rather than talk. I've spoken to a number of women who split from their partners in the first five years of parenthood – the zone of madness! – and desperately regretted it. You wrote about this in *The Making of Love*, which is, I think, my favourite book of yours.

SB: Great! I'll tell Shaaron, because she wrote a lot of that book. At the time, lots of our friends were divorcing, and *The Making of Love* was a real reaction to that. Because painful parts of a marriage are a really important part of growth, both individual and for the relationship. And people mistake it for incompatibility, you know? They think: "We're screwed! We don't get on!" Not realizing that it's like a tectonic plate shifting to allow for a new formation. You always need support for life's changes, and our culture doesn't support hanging in through the tough times. The length of weddings in cultures is proportionate to how long they last, so Indian weddings can last three weeks. But in the West, we're down to half an hour. The time investment is interesting, because it means that other people are involved – you know, "Hey, we're in this wedding, too, and we'll slap your head if you don't work at it!" Love is a team effort, work for a community.

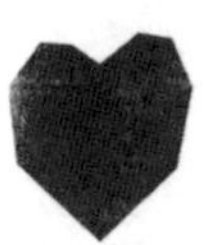

Language and behaviour

The first bite

In moments of sanity, I recognized exactly how little and fragile she is.

From the time of Bethesda's birth, we continually amended basic routines to suit her evolution – from milky hibernation to all-day wakefulness, with dinner followed by a bath followed by stories. One day when she was about two, I lay with her in my arms, which is how she always fell asleep. She generally chattered before beginning to snore, but this night was different: she bit me so violently that she left a bruise.

"I don't want to go to sleep!" she announced.

And tried to bite me again.

I had never been angry with her before, but this time, rage engulfed me. My arm was aching where she had bitten me. I wanted – and this shocked me – to wallop her on the bottom ("How do you like them apples?"). Instead, I grabbed her and firmly pushed my hand against her nappy. "Do not bite Mama", I said through my teeth. She was sitting up – I could see her silhouette in the darkness – and inclined her head. "Bite Dadda?" "No", I said, "do not bite Dadda". "Bite Jacob?" she asked of her best friend. Evidently, she was desperate to sink her fangs into someone, anyone.

"Biting is bad", I said.

The emotional discord of this evening stayed with us for days. When she looked at me, her eyes held a new wariness, and even when she smiled, the smile was quick and not the usual expanse of heart. For the first time ever, she preferred her father. She would grow annoyed when we played, and began to act up. Bethesda had never been anything but the most level-headed of babies, considerate and funny and loving, which is why the shift was so startling. "I want to play with the jigsaw", she would say, and then, when I opened the jigsaw, she would want a book, or jelly or Mr Potato Head or *KerPlunk!* Working not to reinforce negative behaviour, I did not react but instead grew increasingly more wooden as she poured glass after glass of milk on the floor, stopped sleeping by herself and expected to be fed by me or Alex at every meal.

I felt less persecuted when she bit Alex hard on the chest one night as he embraced her, but he was also mystified as to why this was happening. Bethesda had only ever thrown a handful of tantrums, and whilst that caterwauling sometimes reached a pitch only audible to dogs, it was always brief and easily dissolved by an embrace.

It was evident that she felt overwhelmed by emotion – from a distance, the speed and magnitude of her reactions seemed like the sort of breakdown Britney Spears once entertained on a daily basis – but the source of her emotional discord was unclear. "The Terrible Twos" seemed too facile an explanation. She wasn't feverish or teething (formerly the sole causes of late-night psychoses), and there had been no unusual stressors or disruptions to her domestic routine. She owned a small library of books she loved, had wonderful toys, was warm and clean and well-fed, and never watched television. We had a policy of never raising voices in the house, praised her for all good turns, lavishly expressed affection, and had never abused her.

Which is, perhaps, why her anger was so strangely wounding.

We began to increase her sense of power over the world by giving her choices, if never between more than two options lest she become confused. Did she want tortellini or couscous? Would she prefer to read *The Flying Bed* or *Through the Tempests Dark and Wild*?

This technique helped, but she still paced the house like a caged lion.

I sat with her in the afternoons, drawing or making paper flowers – oriental poppies, sweetpeas – but she was restless and slid away from me to visit her father, who was writing in the other room, or to play with a piece of plastic on the floor. My feelings of rejection struck me as ridiculous – in moments of sanity, I recognized exactly how little and fragile she was, and how annoying it must be to be perpetually supervised and organized by the narcissistic apes we call adults – but I was also irritated by her restiveness, and remember daydreaming of growing wings.

After two weeks of her uncharacteristic behaviour, I rang the friend with whom I have shared my deepest feelings about motherhood. She asked me if anything had changed in Bethesda's life. "Nothing!" I cried. "I just wish Jacob would return, because the time we spend together would relieve some of the pressure." "When did he leave?" she asked. "Two weeks –" And then I stopped, realizing that Bethesda's misbehaviour had started the day Jacob had left for vacation. My passionate little girl was not only grieving for her friend, she was disoriented by this grief. Where was he really and why had he left her?

I realized that Bethesda had already lost a number of friends – Holly, whom she had spent significant time with on holiday, and the three adored daughters of a friend who had relocated to a different city. To add to this catalogue of losses would be unimaginably painful for her, and also difficult as she had no point of reference. And so I held and kissed my grieving baby, and assured her that her best friend would soon be home.

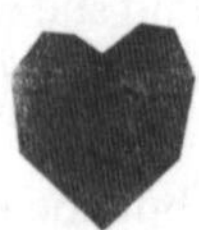

Love in practice

A conversation with Lysa Parker

Our brains develop in the context of relationships.

For twenty years, Lysa Parker has gracefully steered Attachment Parenting International, the non-profit organization she co-founded with her friend and fellow special ed teacher, Barbara Nicholson, into the public consciousness. The bond between the two women has been both enduring and fruitful. *Attached at the Heart: Eight Proven Parenting Principles for Raising Connected and Compassionate Children* is their latest salvo in the war against the neglect and normative abuse of children. In it, Parker, now sixty-three, and Nicholson cite the five protective factors against child abuse and neglect: nurturing and attachment; parenting and child development education; parental resilience; social connections; and concrete supports for parents. It is a beautiful book, pragmatic, heartfelt and charged with hope. Parker, who has comforted thousands by telephone, Skype and face-to-face sessions through her consultancy, parentslifeline.com, has dedicated her life to helping others become more loving in their parenting. "The secret is awareness", she says in that warm, sweet, low Alabama drawl. Her own journey began with an incomplete attachment to her alcoholic mother, a trial that also taught her organization and responsibility. Awarded a bachelor's degree in Education and a master's degree in Human Development and Family Studies, Parker became a Certified Family Life Educator and trained as a facilitator for the Nurturing Parenting Program. Her own experience of motherhood (two sons, a stepdaughter and twin grandsons) and years of teaching troubled children – some with multiple handicaps and/or learning disabilities –

evolved into a grander philosophy of love. Parenting, Parker emphasizes, is the prevention model for societal violence. "Because each of us", she says, "has the potential to change the course of our familial inheritance".

AGB: Before pregnancy, I wanted a caesarean – the idea of a natural birth disgusted me. I had a corrosive relationship with my mother, no sisters, most of my friends were male, and demand-feeding struck me as ludicrous.

LP: That sounds very similar to me! My parents had been spanking parents – typical for their day. I did not have a really good relationship with my mother, either. She passed away at the age of forty-seven. The next year, I had my first son. I had no extended family other than two younger brothers, who didn't live near me and wouldn't have been helpful anyway. As a special ed teacher, I knew a lot about cognitive milestones and behaviour modification. I felt that I was probably more prepared to be a mother than most, because I had all this education. My son quickly turned that around – I realized that I didn't know anything! Looking back at it now, I see that so many of the struggles I experienced were because of my own misinformation and resistance to his needs, and fear of spoiling, and all of that. And then I began attending La Leche League meetings.

AGB: And a metamorphosis took place?

LP: It did. I learned about attachment parenting. This was thirty-four years ago. I made the mistake of waiting until my son arrived – I should have gone to the meetings before; I would have saved myself – and him! – a lot of difficulties. I just didn't know what I was doing. Attending La Leche League meetings made me look at children in a different way, and I was able to watch and observe other mothers with their children. I quickly learned that we should be respectful of our children, and that we need to learn to listen to them and attend to their needs as much as possible.

AGB: Tell me more about your relationship with your mother.

LP: There was alcohol involved. She was an alcoholic, and felt competitive with me. But now I understand that she [had been] living in a war zone in her own family. She was sexually abused. Her sister was sexually abused. Her father was mean and violent, and pretty much drove all his children out of the house. She developed cancer. And then, for the first time, I saw her sober, but it was just too late. I still wish we had had more time to talk through some things. I think she felt a lot of guilt.

AGB: How did she make you feel as a child?

LP: Alone. I kind of withdrew into my own world. I did a lot of reading, got involved in dance, but pretty much kept to myself. I was a sad child. When I look back at pictures, I didn't smile a lot and if I did smile, it looked fake. I just couldn't wait to get out of the house. I felt like an indentured slave. I did a lot of babysitting so that she could have the freedom to do what she wanted. She did spank me a lot, because that was the only tool she had. But again, I wish we could have had time to make amends. From an objective standpoint, I think: well, you know, she did better than her parents did. It wasn't what I would have wanted, it wasn't perfect, but it wasn't as bad as she had endured. It was really sad that when she died, I didn't cry.

AGB: Not an uncommon situation. Some people don't even go to their mother's funeral.

LP: That's very sad.

AGB: It is, but there's a line you can cross as a parent. At a certain point, we all have to take responsibility for our pasts and make amends. Lies kill. Look at our suicide rates.

LP: That's very true of our justice system here [in the United States], where we have violent children who have suffered violent abuse for years, and yet the system's best answer is to try them as adults, put them in prison and throw away the key. The parents are never held accountable. And anybody who has ever tried to talk about these issues – brain damage from abuse, and so on – is told by the prosecution that they're using the "abuse excuse" or just trying to get them off. They belittle therapists and research scientists. Author and neurologist Jonathan Pincus tested and interviewed maybe a couple of hundred violent criminals, including serial killers. When he interviewed these men, they invariably denied they had been abused, and if they had been spanked or beaten, they would say that they deserved it.

AGB: They had internalized the abuser's mindset.

LP: Absolutely! And some even idolized their parents, just like Hitler idolized his. But Pincus didn't stop there. He went deeper. He started interviewing their family members, neighbours, relatives, anyone who knew the child and the family. He discovered that not only were all these violent criminals abused as children, but they were the worst abused of the children in the family. You cannot believe that anyone would treat a human being the way these children were treated.

AGB: As a culture, we need to start understanding violent, antisocial, unruly or pathologically timid behaviour in children as a red flag indicating domestic trouble, rather than punishing them. We need to intervene, and rapidly. Parents need to be hauled up and interviewed.

LP: I can't believe that when a violent murder occurs, we still wail, "What happened?"

AGB: Despite all the evidence, we persist in perceiving violence in children as naughtiness, obstinacy or sinfulness rather than as trauma. Why?

LP: Sir Richard Bowlby, the son of attachment research pioneer John Bowlby, said that looking into the mirror at one's own attachment can be so upsetting that we turn away from it, you know? People who were ineptly or inadequately nurtured as an infant cannot witness a baby being nurtured and loved and cared for without having unimaginable pain triggered in them – it's just too frightening for them, re-experiencing those feelings.

AGB: Which is why an increasing number of people find babies and the nurturance of babies – in particular, breastfeeding – so disturbing. I mean, they're really confronted by it.

LP: Exactly!

AGB: The corollary is, of course, the overlooking of child abuse.

I remember walking along a promenade with a friend. It was a beautiful day, there were hundreds of people milling about. And a woman walked past, berating her four or so year-old son with language I never thought it was possible to use with a child. I mean, it was just horrendous. And nobody said a word. I turned to my friend, a financier. "Just ignore it", he said. Not one person stood up for this little boy. Had a man addressed a woman in this fashion, some other man would have intervened. But because it was a little child, no-one said anything, including me. And so I just stared the mother down but said nothing. I still wonder whether that boy made it to manhood. My conscience pricks. Because I failed him. Every adult walking on that promenade that day failed him. And I have never forgiven myself. Because the people who stand by and do nothing when a child is being abused are just as accountable as the abuser. By saying nothing, I contributed to that boy's abuse.

LP: When we're under stress, we go to flight, fight or freeze. You froze.

AGB: All of us – even those of us who don't have children – have to protect children, if only to protect that which children represent: innocence, vulnerability, tenderness.

LP: We are all responsible – they are all our children.

AGB: But what can you do when you see someone abusing a little child? What's the protocol?

LP: That kind of situation is so common. I could've said something, I should've said something … but I didn't. A widespread not-knowing-what-to-say. The accepted advice is this: don't become confrontational towards an abusive parent, but show them empathy. Intervene to stop what's going on by changing the subject, saying something kind to the child, showing empathy for the parent's tiredness. You could go up and say something like, "You sound really frustrated," or "You seem to be having a hard time – is there anything I can do to help? I'm a parent, too". Just sharing how overwhelming it can be to be a parent. Offer to help. Suspend judgment. And if they turn on you, say: "I understand you're upset, but I'm here to help you. Is there anything I can do? Please let me help." It would be good to come up with a strategy. The main thing is to show empathy first.

AGB: You became aware of an explosion of violence in children in the early nineties.

LP: I did. I'd gone back to teaching, and had the children no-one else wanted. They had learning disabilities, sure, but they also had a lot of emotional problems, and they dated back to kindergarten. I became very disturbed about that. Their lives could have been so different had someone intervened. Because it was my observation that their issues were due to poor parenting.

AGB: A psychiatrist from a US children's detention centre wrote to me about *The Eclipse*, the book I wrote about my brother's suicide. "I still find it difficult to understand why these children are in here", she wrote, "because the people who should be in here are their parents. These children are all victims. And the system has failed them."

LP: Mine were seventh and eighth grade students. I had a thirteen-year-old student who was a father already, another who was trying to initiate into a gang, and then I had a female student whose father used to play her porno movies. There was so much inappropriate behaviour, the saying of inappropriate things. I've had children masturbate in class. As Alice Miller would say, I was their enlightened witness, an oasis of stability. I really tried to give them a safe place, but they would still break into fights. They were angry. One boy was giving me a hard time and I couldn't deal with it, so I sent him to the principal. I had no idea that they were going to paddle [spank] him; of course it made no difference. When you're brutalized all the time at home, more violence just doesn't matter. And so I thought: I will never do that again. It was heartbreaking for me. And that was part of the impetus for Barbara and me starting Attachment Parenting International. Attachment parenting had changed us so much as mothers, as women, and we wanted to give back. We just felt like it was the key.

AGB: Children are mirrors. This was never brought home to me until I had my own daughter. Children are always scapegoated for their parents' inadequacies – in part, because the sense of guilt can be intolerable. Hence the externalisation, because the ability to confront guilt head-on is rare. I failed: not an easy statement to make in this PR-saturated culture. And yet acknowledgment of wrongdoing is critical to our children's mental health, absolutely critical.

LP: Exactly! Parents feel shame, and try to deflect that by blaming the shame. In *Parenting from the Heart*, we talk about the importance of self-reflection. When you're pregnant – or even before you have children – you need to talk to your partner about the way you were raised, and your feelings about that, and how you want to raise your child, and what kinds of strategies do you not want to use with your child. Because we all have wounds, and children will bring out those wounds if they're not healed. I'm still working on mine. Mindfulness is an important lesson. Remaining in the present moment. Learning how to reframe your perceptions and language. Basically, we need to learn how to stay in the prefrontal cortex. We can learn to sidestep the part of the brain that stores all those bad memories and all those traumas. It's a lifelong process, but the first step is awareness.

AGB: I've seen a whole spectrum of behaviour in mothers. I've seen what I call avoidant mothers, who almost entirely delegate mothering; I've seen mothers who passionately love their children but are emotionally dislocated and uninformed, creating ambivalence in their children. I've seen many mothers hijacked by the unexamined heart. One mother I know, a woman who deeply loves her toddler son, told me that she had once ground a key into the back of his hand when he wouldn't stop misbehaving; the thing that scared her, she said, was that she had enjoyed it. So many mothers who, because of a lack of marital, family and community support, are quietly imploding: they do not know how to cope. Mothering is such a big job, and so sacred. There is nothing more relevant to the human condition, nothing. And yet the neurobiology of human evolution isn't taught in schools.

LP: There would be a lot of resistance from teachers. They're so focused on testing – teaching to the test, standardized testing – so it's hard to get any new information in the curriculum.

AGB: I find this extraordinary, as parenthood is the lynchpin of civilization.

LP: That's right.

AGB: Now, you've described our culture as toxic to children. Can you tell me more about that?

LP: There were studies done in 2001 or thereabouts on families who had emigrated to the United States. On arrival, the children were deemed emotionally healthy, and the families were going well. But after one generation, the families ended up having all kinds of issues that are typical of American families – this is typical of enculturation – and so their rates of mental illness, suicide and violence all increased to that of the national norm. Western culture is poisoned. Children don't feel valued in this culture. They did a survey of middle school students and found that only 20 per cent of them felt that adults cared about them. These children don't feel connected to their families, they don't feel connected to their communities. As human beings we have this drive to have a family, and if we don't have a cohesive family we'll seek out another family, which might be a gang, or unsavoury characters who lead children down the path of drugs and addiction.

AGB: I find the issue of addiction interesting because all addiction is a yearning for transcendence. And I found that very transcendence in mothering Bethesda, because love is transcendence.

LP: Absolutely.

AGB: In our culture, we're conditioned to understand that in order to survive, we must be selfish. We're bamboozled into achieving and producing without any consideration of the cost – not only to others, but to ourselves. And it's such a lie. Co-operation and service are the bases of a functional civilization. Our focus on material success is antiquated, patriarchal.

LP: Yes, instead of embracing our femininity. The patriarchal perspective is reflected in the lack of maternity leave and paternity leave, and in the lack of child-friendly, family-friendly policies. It's reflected in the model of birth that we have … which is the beginning of a woman's journey that, if done correctly, can truly enhance the attachment relationship and empower her.

AGB: You've spoken about how disconnection is endemic in our culture …

LP: We have to hold onto our children despite what society tells us, despite this pathological need for teaching our children to be independent and pushing them away. We have to work on ways to stay connected and give them the freedom to return if they need to. It takes a lot of effort. You have to be their advocate from before birth. Once they begin school, you have to protect them from all the forces that are going to be aimed at them. Schools don't care about the child–parent connection. We have to protect our children from consumerism, from advertising, television, the internet.

AGB: It's rare for children to have unbroken communication with their mothers any more. We're too distracted to hold their hands and teach them about the world. I made a conscious choice to block the cacophony out years ago. I hardly ever even bother answering the phone any more.

LP: I've known families who can't sleep without the TV running all night. It's just another form of addiction. You need to change those things that aren't working for you and get peace back into your life. Building a support network of like-minded women is essential. Because it's like you were saying earlier, our children mirror us. Our brains develop in the context of relationships. So when a child is disorganized, can't control overwhelming feelings, or seems angry or sad, it's time to look at the relationship – you know, what is it about the relationship that is not going well? I love the metaphor of a flower. Say you have a potted flower. It was doing well, but all of a sudden, it's starting to wilt and the leaves are browning. So do we blame the plant? Or do we say, "What does that plant need? Am I giving it too much water or not enough? Is it getting enough sunlight?"

AGB: Part of the issue is that so many of us don't know our children well enough to distinguish any divergence from their norm. Most of us work big hours. Most children attend school. Many attend daycare. And then they come home and watch TV or go on Facebook, just as we do. In short, those who should know us most deeply are strangers. I mean, I've known laundromat owners better than I knew my own father! We're sacrificing love and intimacy to pursue status and entertainment.

LP: Biology drives children to seek attachment to the primary caregiver. There are a lot of reasons for that. Initially, the child has imprinted the mother's voice, the mother's smell, her pheromones. And there's also something going on with the brain: neural resonance. By having a relationship with one person, the infant brain develops a healthier pattern. The problem with having multiple caregivers, a situation we call caregiver roulette, is that the child has no neural resonance with anyone. There's nothing familiar. Infants and young children thrive best in intimate, loving, consistent relationships, and they're not getting that if they're going from caregiver to caregiver.

AGB: I remember staggering around with Bethesda – the birth had wrecked my lower back – feeling like the luckiest woman in the world … in this disastrous apartment, on the brink of bankruptcy, and 20 kilos overweight. In retrospect, it was hilarious.

LP: Society makes it hard for mothers to fall in love with their babies. If they have to go back to work, they start distancing themselves, even when the baby is in utero. They think: I don't want to become too attached, because I have to go back to work. I have to steel myself! I have to compartmentalize my feelings because I have to go back to work. We know that a mother's stress or depression cause babies and children great anxiety, but what I would like to see is mothers educated about how blissful a relationship with a baby can be. Some women have Freudian fears, you know – if they get that close to their children it might stir sexual feeling. You know: Why co-sleep? Why breastfeed for long periods of time? It must be you! You must have some kind of weird need!

AGB: One woman I know refused to breastfeed because she perceived her breasts as exclusively sexual. So her newborns didn't even get colostrum, which contains antibodies against disease. One media personality memorably said that the very thought made her feel "really funny". What I don't understand is why these women continue to kiss their husbands with the same mouth they use to vomit.

LP: [laughs] Our culture sexualizes women, which is why our breasts are sexualized. And the fact that women implicitly accept this sexualization shows you how bad the situation still is. Part of our evolution as a culture – and I think we are evolving – is evidenced in the fact that thirty years ago, to talk about a child nursing for a year was shocking. And now we're saying it's okay to breastfeed for two. The more this is talked about it, the more doors open. It makes people think.

AGB: So what can fathers do?

LP: Fathers need to realize that they are the gatekeepers for the mother. A father needs to allow his partner the opportunity to get to know her baby while keeping well-meaning friends and family at bay. A woman needs to learn how to hold her baby and feed him and connect with him. Too often, everyone descends en masse to celebrate, but those first thirty days should be sacred. Which is not to say that grandparents can't come see the baby, but visits need to be limited to immediate family. As a community, we need to support new mothers by taking meals. My daughter-in-law had a baby six weeks ago, so I am doing what I teach others to do, and that is: taking her meals, going over and doing housework for her, holding the baby if she needs to take a shower and so on. All mothers need to be nurtured while they're learning to love their babies.

AGB: So what you're saying is that as a culture, we need to not only allow but create the space that allows mothers to bond with their babies. Because that is where the problems begin: when mothers are encouraged to separate from their infants. And it's very cleverly masked. One of my favourites is the new 'get your body back' insanity. As if new mothers don't have more important things to think about. One of the most devoted mothers I knew, an aesthetically beautiful woman, lived on broccoli to regain her figure. Unsurprisingly, her son self-weaned before he was a year old. I mean, if you're taking time out to do sit-ups, not only does that entail a dramatic shift in consciousness from your baby to your waistline, it leeches time and energy from mothering. It trains you to separate. I see so many mothers who walk their babies not to share the experience of the sunlight or talk to them, but to get exercise. They even wear headphones. And the poor baby lies there like a lemon.

LP: [laughs] It's okay to look like a blimp for a year, you know?

AGB: I've also known situations where grandparents actively opposed couples caring for their own children. The idea that caring for your own child is a lifestyle option is so prevalent.

LP: It's such an ignorant perspective.

AGB: And so toxic. I don't think people understand the importance of attachment – they see it as a luxury, essentially unnecessary. It's as if attachment parenting can only be practised by an elite.

LP: Anybody can practise attachment parenting. The media has portrayed it as cookie cutter – you know, you have to breastfeed; you have to wear your baby; you have to bedshare. But attachment parenting is about responsiveness – sensitive responsiveness is the key to attachment theory. If you're a working parent, it's all the more reason to practise attachment parenting. You may not have the ideal situation, but if you can balance the situation with lots of hugs and cuddles and caring, then you and your child are going to be a lot better off. We all have emotional tanks that have to be filled on a regular basis, and when we're away from each other throughout the day, our tanks empty. The best way to fill up your child's emotional tank is to give them your time and that closeness and that reconnection, so that anybody on any economic level in any situation can practise attachment parenting, but they need the awareness. Interactions with children need to be conscious.

AGB: So how do we start respecting children?

LP: It begins by looking at the world through their eyes. That's the golden rule of parenting: treat your child the way you would be treated. As you noted before, they talk about reverence for parents in many religions, but why aren't children included in that? We respect children by seeing who they really are –

as spiritual beings, as human beings, as sacred beings. We respect them through language: how we treat them, how we speak to them, how we interact with them. Children need to see the light come on in your eyes when they enter the room.

Lysa Parker's 8 steps to attachment

1. *Prepare for pregnancy, birth and parenting* Educated parents tend to have less fear and better births when they are actively involved in the process.

2. *Feed with love and respect* Feeding is more than giving your baby nutrition, it's part of the attachment process. Breastfeeding is nature's ideal model for attachment and if you're bottle-feeding, we encourage you to switch sides when feeding and talk to and gaze at your baby.

3. *Respond with sensitivity* This is the most important finding of most attachment research. Sensitive and responsive parents tend to have securely attached children.

4. *Use nurturing touch* Children all need touch, and babies even more so to help them thrive. Holding, babywearing and infant massage are all ways to meet your baby's need for touch.

5. *Ensure safe sleep, physically and emotionally* Parenting is a 24/7 experience. Whether bedsharing or in a separate sleep surface, babies still need to feel in close proximity and in a safe sleep environment. Parents who have no intention of bedsharing with their baby need to prepare their bed "as if". When mum and dad need sleep, studies support that bedsharing offers more sleep and better quality of sleep as well as enhancing the breastfeeding relationship. A more dangerous scenario is for parents to fall asleep in a recliner or on a couch. Attachment Parenting International provides safe sleep guidelines on their website.

6. *Provide consistent, loving care* Babies and young children need consistency of care from a loving, responsive caregiver. Caregiver roulette is damaging to their security of attachment, so if the primary caregiver works outside the home, find a reliable relative, nanny, in-home caregiver or facility with a low adult/child ratio and low turnover of caregivers.

7. *Practise positive discipline* The goal of positive discipline is to maintain the bonds of trust and empathy, while teaching appropriate boundaries. Positive discipline teaches inner discipline rather than discipline that relies on force, coercion, spanking or other forms of punishment.

8. *Strive for balance in your personal and family life* Simplify your life and you will be less stressed, and that includes not over-scheduling. Find time to nurture and nourish your body, mind and spirit, because when parents feel burned out there is nothing left to give our children, spouses or partners. Know that finding balance is a journey, not a destination.

attachmentparenting.org

Waiting for Bethesda

In the dressing room, with roses

It had taken us years to dare to admit to the desire to sometimes be as feminine as it is possible to be.

It was a warm and easy afternoon, that time of day when country towns and certain urban enclaves surrender to a torpor I have always felt was not only somehow magical, but critical to regeneration. As Bethesda and I approached the old church hall through dappled sunlight, she gripped my hand.

"Mama", she asked, "will you stay to watch me?"

Hoisting my big, warm, delicious two-and-a-half-year-old high in my arms, I pressed my forehead to hers. "I'm not allowed to watch", I said, "but I promise I'll wait in the next room".

The ballet school's stern and elegant proprietor forbade mothers from watching lest they distract their toddlers from holding hands in a circle, so we congregated in the dressing room like decadent fin-de-siècle aristocrats hoping to charm the principal artistes after the show (I may have worn a perfumed cravat pinned with a pearl and carried a loose bouquet of peonies).

A rhinoceros could not have dragged me from her orbit.

With hairpins in our mouths, we (the dressing room mothers) all fussed over our daughters' hair until it shone, and then we decorated it with bands and ribbons; in turn, our daughters allowed themselves to be so ornamented, made conscious through maternal service of their own importance. (I have seen the same expressions on the faces of boys whose mothers tie the laces of their football boots, or children whose mothers enthusiastically push them on swings.) Far from lessening our sense of self-value, serving our daughters somehow felt exhilarating, as fulfilling a means of self-expression as that which we found in work. Of what worth, after all, is love without manifestation?

Having inexpertly styled my baby's hair, poured her warm and wriggly puppy body into a pink leotard and a voile skirt, and stuffed those dainty pork-chop feet into ballet shoes, I faltered a little as I watched her take her place among her floral peers – Annabel, Ava, Ruby and all the other girls who sat, grave, erect-backed and with hands in laps, awaiting instruction. Their teacher was a young grandmother in the mould of the French actress and dancer Leslie Caron, lithe in her long black bloomers and instructing her charges to address their bottoms not as bums or butts but derrières. Bethesda loved her.

Shannon, Ava's mother, and I took turns in standing on milk crates to peer in through the windows, but were sprung by the proprietor, who did not take lightly to our disobedience. Chastened, we retreated to the dressing room and, as Chopin drifted in under the door, exchanged recollections of girlhood – Shannon, a working mother who had studied ballet as a girl of six in a leotard that did not fit, and I, who was abandoned to classes in a cold civic hall by a mother eager to escape maternal obligation. It had taken us years to dare to admit to the desire to sometimes be as feminine as it is possible to be, if only within the context of dance – all elongated throats and sweeping arms, lost in a half-lit dream of silk and tulle.

Therein, one of the most outrageously generous gifts of motherhood: the opportunity to heal childhood wounds by changing the inherited parental template. Shannon and I certainly had no interest in propelling our daughters toward the Covent Garden boards, but what we did want is for the needs that had, in us, been frustrated to be satisfied in them. Not all girls have the same needs, but ours did, and we were gratified by watching them revel so openly in their gratification.

My little monkey anticipated each class as if it were the grandest ball. At home, she practised twirling with great intensity, inevitably crashing into occasional tables or walls, and when she did, I could think only of Alan Ball's line from the 1999 film *American Beauty*: "Sometimes there's so much beauty in the world I feel like I can't take it … and my heart is going to cave in."

In that old church hall, Bethesda had her first experience of formal instruction and her first experience of formal femininity. There she also learned the rudiments of socialization: in those preschool ballet lessons, a ceremonial form of female friendship. The girls admired each other's dolls and dresses, learned to take turns in playing Cinderella, and discovered through tribal elders the bond that can be found in shared enterprise. When the teacher marvelled that Bethesda was "entirely devoid of spite" and made a point of stopping to help those who floundered, I felt a pressure on my heart that I laboured to contain.

After a year or so, my husband and I decided that we had had enough of urban decay and relocated to the country. I experienced a surprisingly sharp sorrow at the prospect of enrolling Bethesda in a new class. The sense of community fostered by that church hall school of dance was in itself precious; in cultures fragmented by over-participation in the paid workforce (and here I am referring to that of both sexes), the opportunity to create emotional affinities is rare. Those little girls and the mothers who waited for them in that dressing room represented that which I most love about women: the need for intimacy within the context of grace. Bethesda still misses them, as do I.

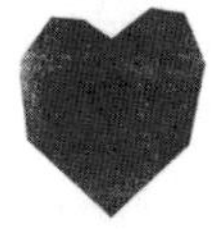

The man who saved my life

Remembering Peter

I kept skipping out on love, picking men who, like me, had only the most cursory capacity for intimacy.

I once suffered from a despair so violent that each day at five I stared out at the evening's encroachment, fearing it would overwhelm all that I understood. Nights could be like that; everything contained during work hours could unravel with disconcerting speed, causing me to feel as if I were holding myself together with willpower alone. The anxiety was terrible. Not infrequently I lay awake until five in the morning, as restless as if I had been lying on hot tin, which, in a way, I was; depression does not only manifest in inertia. It can burn through a life, terrifying sufferers into compulsive distraction. My method of running interference was to work, if only because it suggested the very opposite of listlessness: an appetite for life so voracious that there are never enough hours in the day to do it all.

For years, I worked seven-day weeks, through birthdays and most public holidays, Christmases and New Year's Eves included. I worked mornings and afternoons, resuming work after dinner. I remember feeling as if life were a protracted exercise in pulling myself out of a well by a rope, and that rope was work. Many friends laboured equally hard to disguise their dark internal worlds, camouflaging histories of addiction, incest, mental illness, promiscuity, traumatic bereavement and violence: life as a charade. The suicides were especially compelling, because that is where their stories ended and our stories of bereavement began. Rapidly, they ran into double figures: the first boy who ever kissed me; an infinitely kind gay colleague; my outwardly successful brother. Ironically, the most emotionally damaged were, in my experience, the most influential; part of the damage is a belief that being "ordinary" – unclouded, uncomplicated – is to be lesser.

In our circle, stress was a valuable status marker: I stress, therefore I am. To us, stress carried the suggestion of responsibility, desirability, clout. And everyone I knew was always stressed. Nobody had time for anything unrelated to status, it seemed – even children were sidelined, and relationships were derailed by the pressure. The weddings I attended were outnumbered by divorces, and most of the relationships I knew were crippled by infidelity, indifference, compulsion. In this respect, I was a little different; I kept skipping out on love, picking men who, like me, had only the most cursory capacity for intimacy. It was easier to date and then, citing my partner's intolerable incompetence, leave them after a few weeks, than it was to admit that I had no idea what I was doing.

I had created a protective false self, and was rewarded for that false self; and I related almost exclusively through that self until the falsity itself became asphyxiating.

The turning point in my consciousness was when I walked out on my fiancé. On my return home, I realized – not for the first time, but with new gravity – that I really needed help. Yes, almost every man I had ever dated was spectacularly dysfunctional – or, as I then romantically perceived it, "tormented" – but I was the common denominator, and it was time to accept responsibility for my choices. For years, I had used these fractured men to justify my cynicism and workaholism, and the grief, insomnia and casual anorexia were no longer of any interest to me. I was tired of feeling as if nothing other than the opinions of people I did not even like mattered. I wanted to return to the self I had abandoned, the girl I was before the fall, unfettered by insult, free.

To this end, I began scouting for a therapist. Over the course of a single meeting, one decided that I was "just like Dorothy Parker"; the next, a man with pressed slacks and a gimlet stare, expressed more interest in the biochemical impact of prescription drugs than in any detail of my life; the third, a woman with an array of macramé pot-plant holders suspended from the ceiling, was so universal – and, concomitantly, impersonal – in her compassion that I felt as if I were having an audience with the Dalai Lama. But Peter, the psychiatrist who saved my life, actually listened, and the memory of our first session can still exhilarate me.

"You're very angry", he quietly said. "I can help you with that".

I consulted Peter for seven years – sometimes twice a week, and with an eighteen-month break. To the surprise of certain friends, the fact that I had a therapist never struck me as odd or damning – the opposite, in fact; like Tony Soprano and Woody Allen's Alvy Singer, I was captivated by the situation's unique intimacies. I was also curious. Who would I be when I quit? And what would surface in the interim?

There were times when I would sob until I shook, until my eyelids were so swollen that it pained me to open them, and through hiccoughs, trembling, I would hiss, "Don't touch me!" as he moved to place a gentle hand on my shoulder. There were times when we seemed locked into our chairs, discrete, the static between us more eloquent than words. But there was never a moment when I doubted Peter's ability to heal me.

When he moved his practice to a bungalow adjacent to a private eating disorders hospital in a distant suburb, I followed – catching two buses and a train and walking for twenty minutes – at times through hail, at times through rain – to see him, and then, because of train schedules, waiting for half an hour in the garden, where I would sit, lost in the green music of unseen tennis games behind the camphor laurels. There I smoked a thousand cigarettes, and there I dreamed like a child dreams, and there I felt entirely unassailable.

Inside, Peter, upright and angular, in blue and white, would focus – or so I felt – on a point in me immune to chaos, a core untouched by suffering or fear, a self he somehow discerned beneath the rage and devastation. I had never before known what it was to be the focal point of sustained caring. Initially, it was uncomfortable, and then it felt like coming home. In 1998, Israeli researchers working with a beam of electrons discovered that the very act of observation changes the nature of the observed – the more prolonged the focus, the greater the observer's influence on the observed: the quantum physics behind my psychic revolution. Gradually, I began to see myself not through the jaundiced eyes of my parents, but through his: valuable not for obedience or achievement, but for elementary being. Through him, I actually began to like myself.

The magic Peter worked cannot be attributed to a formula, and no antidepressants were involved. It was an amalgam of factors – his non-directive, rather than instructional, approach; patience; honesty; basic compatibility; faith and, ultimately, love. Because notwithstanding necessary professional standardization, the best therapy is all about love.

In time, the sense of urgency that characterized our early sessions faded to a jovial familiarity, and that is when I knew our work together had been done. Unlike Lot's wife, I no longer wanted to look back; for the first time, the future struck me as far more intriguing. The frequency of our consultations changed from once a week to once a fortnight, and then from once a fortnight to once a month, until it became obvious that I was coping – if not perfectly, then well enough. Life was good, and I was alright, too.

We remained in touch, if not exactly as friends; there is no parity between us. Peter's authority is parental in scope – while he knows everything about me, I know almost nothing about him other than his passion for his wife, three brilliant daughters and scuba diving. When, in an email, he casually mentioned a love of jazz, I was floored. Jazz? This made me realize how limited patients need their therapists to be in order to regenerate. The Peter I knew belonged in a swivel chair, against a backdrop of magnolia paint and banal prints. There is no room in that portrait for jazz. I still don't know if I am ready for him to exist in three dimensions. And, in that respect, he is like a mother; while I am aware that he exists outside his rooms, part of me will always want him to myself.

Because therapists can refine understanding with a clarity and impartiality absent in families or friendship, I still sporadically seek their counsel. I have, since ending therapy, consulted psychologists who specialize in relevant areas, a practice I regard as psychic spot-welding. Addictions expert Sky, who – in flowing silks and with hair like panned gold in the sun – helped me kick a two-pack-a-day habit; John, the enigmatic, chain-smoking forensic counsellor who guided me through the aftermath of my brother's suicide; Nichola, the infinitely tender maternal-infant counsellor who, when I was sickened with guilt after my baby was burned by a shaft of late sunlight, somehow made me laugh.

I no longer remember what it is to feel incapable. However formidable the crisis, I now know that I will cope. I continue to work with carnivorous ease, but also luxuriate in time spent with my husband and our luminous daughter. For the first time in my life, I revel in cooking, eating, sleep. I make time to listen to the rain. In every sense, I tend to this, my garden. And somewhere in a city, there is a man – upright, angular, in blue and white – teaching another person how to want to live. My gratitude to him is immortal.

An angel at my table

A conversation with Laura Markham

Your children will cry when you show empathy.

Laura Markham is rapidly evolving into one of the world's best-loved parenting experts. Her website, ahaparenting.com, is an invaluable resource for mothers interested in changing destructive, unrewarding or uninspiring dynamics with their children. A clinical psychologist, Markham, fifty-eight, is now a parenting coach and author of the profoundly wise *Peaceful Parent, Happy Kids: How to Stop Yelling and Start Connecting* (in my review of the book, I noted that a copy should be given to every mother along with her newborn). At the core of Markham's work: connection and parental responsibility. Connection because there is no co-operation without it, and responsibility because the only way any child can be taught to regulate its emotions is by parental example. She believes that as a culture, we need to move beyond the idea of punishment if only because it erodes the parent–child bond; instead, she encourages parents to set limits with generosity and empathy. "What about families that begin punishing their toddler?" she asks. "They're pushing their little one away each time, and lessening their influence on their child without even knowing it. As long as we can scare her and drag her into 'time out', our child may obey our directives. But her willingness to listen to us diminishes with every punishment, and by the time she's five or six and too big to physically control, her attitude will be rebellious. This will continue to escalate." Markham serves as an expert for Mothering.com and numerous other websites. She has been featured on the Fox Morning Show, CNN, and extensively on radio, and her insightful daily newsletter has over 30,000 subscribers (I am one). A long-married mother of two, Markham has alchemized a grief-filled childhood into a philosophy that is helping to transform our world for the better, child by child.

AGB: As a mother, I've found that my flashpoint is exhaustion.

LM: Everyone's flashpoint is exhaustion!

AGB: When I'm tired, I catch myself saying the most idiotic things to my daughter – "That's it! I'm giving your dolls' house away to charity!" Desperate, stupid things. And when our exhaustions collide, when she's tired, too, it's a conflagration of idiocy. You often speak about the importance of taking time out, but it's not always possible. Sometimes, I find there's just too much on.

LM: It is really, really hard to have a lot of responsibilities and be a good parent at the same time. Preventative maintenance works best, but if you're having a really busy week, you're not going to have time for preventative maintenance, so the children will act up more, right? The price of a busy week is losing it as a parent. And if you find yourself with busy week followed by busy week, it's a signal that there's something wrong with your life and some hard choices have to get made.

AGB: After I hit flashpoint, I always apologize to Bethesda. "I am so sorry that I yelled, Bunny. I'm so tired today, and just feeling overwhelmed. Please forgive me for being such a complete idiot. You didn't deserve it." And she's good at it, too. Often, she'll come up after a disagreement and say, "Let's be friends" or "I'm sorry for yelling, Mama – I took out all my stress from school today on you".

LM: That is wonderful. I would add that you don't have to be perfect. Your daughter learns a lot by seeing that a relationship can have a disruption and that you can make up afterward. If we are to teach our children to have loving and rewarding relationships, then they need to see those relationships in their full breadth, which includes the inevitable rifts that happen in any relationship. They need to see that two people who love each other can disagree, or can even at times hurt each other: that there can be a rift, and that it can be repaired. And when we apologize to our children, we're modelling that reparation, so I think it's critical to apologize. I would add that if you find yourself apologizing on a frequent basis to your child, then you undermine your credibility. In that case, you have to ask yourself why you're under such stress and what you can do to change it.

AGB: Laura, I have to take this opportunity to thank you for literally saving my sanity during one of the most difficult years of my life. I was under an avalanche of stress – two consecutive deaths in the immediate family, terrible debt, oppressive work commitments, eight months of serious illness, three house moves, intrafamilial legal issues, my husband's sustained depression after unsupportable GFC-related losses … I mean, it was the perfect storm. Picking up on my stress, Bethesda began having problems falling asleep. So I'd put her to bed and try to work – I only worked for four hours during the day when my husband minded her and at night, while she slept – and she'd creep out of bed and start tearing around the house. This would happen repeatedly – not every night, but often. She also had a heightened sensitivity to salicylates, so despite a very strict diet – only proteins and carbohydrates after 2 pm – some would slip through and keep her awake. You can imagine the stress; I mean, I actually remember my scalp prickling from the tension. I was responsible for holding everything together and my physical health began to deteriorate. And so I cracked, and began to spank her when she didn't stay in her room. Which drove me to the point of madness – the guilt was intolerable – as I had never even raised my voice with her before she turned four.

LM: Most parents exhaust themselves and then lash out, knowing it's not the way they want to parent but at that moment, they're in a rage. The most effective thing we can do at such moments is to STOP. Literally just stop: shut your mouth, walk away. You may need to leave the room. Of course, it's harder with your child, because a child can freak out when you leave the room. Situations such as the running-around-the-house thing aren't going to get solved in a night; they need a little time, probably a month. But you can stop yourself from losing it.

AGB: I didn't have a month – I literally did not have one. There were two contracts to fulfil, debts to pay: I'd overcommitted myself, because my husband was suffering from a clinical depression. One night after spanking her, I broke down. I was so enraged, I actually chased her around the house. And she turned to look at me, and said – I will never forget this – "You think you're teaching me when you spank me, but all you're doing is making me angry."

LM: Wow.

AGB: [crying] I've always trained Bethesda to articulate her needs – to understand that her feelings are her own. This little person held a mirror up to me, and I was horrified. And so I actually prayed for help for the first time in what? Three decades? Because I no longer knew what to do. The one golden thing in my life was this child, and I was failing her. And then I went online and found you. And here we are, years later, talking about that night. Everything changed from that moment on.

LM: Discipline and punishment undermine trust. Imagine if you had a relationship with your husband where you did something he didn't like, and he said: "That's it, then! I'm going to give your favourite such-and-such away." or "I'm going to put you over my knee and spank you!" We need to look at children as people. I remember being stood in the corner by my stepmother. When I was allowed to come out, she'd ask, "What did you learn?", and I'd parrot back what I was expected to learn. You know, I remember nothing of what she taught me, but I do remember this: I was livid at her, and spent the whole time I was standing in the corner thinking what a horrible person she was and how I would never, ever, ever make it up with her. I resented her for years and years and years. And she would give me a hug afterward. I hear this from parents all the time – "I send them to the corner and give them a hug and then it's all fine!" And I think: "Well, maybe your child's different from the way I was, but with most normal kids, that's not how it's going to work!"

AGB: What are children really doing when they misbehave?

LM: When a child misbehaves he is acting out in feelings what he cannot articulate in words. A baby has no words, so it cries. But even a preschooler who has words can whine or just go off and hit the baby when they don't know how to express the way they feel in words.

AGB: So what are they feeling when they misbehave?

LM: Fear, mostly. Small humans often feel fear. As they don't know what to do with that fear or pain, they save it up for a time when they feel safe. Sometimes, of course, the feeling has just arisen in that moment, from what's going on in the home, and sometimes, like your daughter, they're picking up on our feelings. Children pick up feelings so quickly, particularly if they're connected.

AGB: One of the life-changing suggestions you make to parents who have lost the plot is to play what you call the Fix Game, which was a turning point in my relationship with Bethesda. Allow me to quote from your website: "Remind her how much you love her by playing the Fix Game. You play the bumbler as you chase her, hug, kiss, let her get away and repeat again and again: 'I need my Chelsea fix … You can't get away … I have to hug you and cover you with kisses … oh, no, you got away … I'm coming after you … I just have to kiss you more and hug you more …'"

LM: The Fix Game is designed to fix whatever's wrong with your child. The problem is usually that your child doesn't feel connected or loved, and so the Fix Game is simply acting out that love with your child in a way that gets your child laughing, because the laughter helps release oxytocin, which is the bonding hormone. So as your child bonds with you, she becomes convinced that you really do love her because you're basically say to her, "Oh, I need you! I have to hug you! I have to cover you with kisses! Oh, no – you got away! I'm coming after you! Why are you so fast? Why are you so strong? You always get away from me! No! I'm going to get you!" And you catch them, and you hug them, and then they get away again and you do it again, and if you have two parents, you can even fight over the child – "Oh, you always get to hug her! I want to hug her!" And then she feels that even though there's a new baby, or mummy yelled at her last night: "Yes, indeed: I am loved."

AGB: Now tell me a little bit about your own childhood.

LM: Okay. My father, Emerson Markham, comes from a long line of readers. Books are a big thing in our family. He worked for the Federal Government his entire life – for the Peace Corps, the Veterans Administration, and Vista, the Corporation for National and Community Service.

AGB: A giver, in other words.

LM: Absolutely! One of the best things he used to say was: "You've been blessed with parents who love you, enough to eat, a good brain, and you need to use that to make the world a better place."

AGB: I tell Bethesda that it is her destiny to be happy, because it's possible to be happy even in the most terrible of circumstances.

LM: He thinks like that, too. Off and on, my mother took me to a Unitarian-Universalist church. I remember learning about the Vietnam War and how bad it was, and the civil rights movement and how good it was. There was no talk of God or Jesus; there was no Christianity in that church at all.

AGB: Do you have siblings?

LM: Yes, I have a lot of siblings! I have two brothers, one older and one younger, and then my parents divorced and they each remarried. My mother and stepfather had one son, who's twelve years younger than I am, and I was very much involved with raising him for the first few years of his life. He slept in my room, I was very attached to him. I learned some of the first lessons about parenting from being his big sister. My dad, whom I did not live with but saw every other weekend, remarried, and he and my stepmother had two daughters and a son.

AGB: Seven children?!

LM: Between three marriages. I was the only fourth grader I knew whose parents were divorced.

AGB: That must have been just before the big wave of divorces.

My generation was swept away. It was chaotic, a social experiment. You've said that you didn't feel loved by your mother.

LM: My father had good parents and was able to parent me very well, but my mother did not. Her mother told her that she was an accident; they had not wanted a child. My mother was a very lonely child and an only child. Her mother protected but did not particularly love her, or at least did not tell her ever that she loved her, or did not act like she loved her. My grandmother, on her death bed, confessed to having had an abortion when she was a young woman, and I think that the experience wounded her so greatly that she was unable to forgive herself and unable to love the child she eventually had. I'm not sure that's the only reason, but it played some role.

AGB: Did your mother favour your brothers?

LM: No! Definitely not. Of the three children in her first marriage, I was her favourite. Later, when my half-brother was born, I think my mother did love him more, but I doted on him to such a degree that I was never jealous of him at all; I felt, in fact, that she wasn't loving him enough. My relationship with him was affected as I left to live with my father and then with some family friends. I found myself unable to live with my stepfather … or my stepmother.

AGB: Was your stepfather sexually abusive?

LM: Yes. He sexually abused me when I was nine and ten years old. I began to cry when he came near me. I would cry in the house. I would cry when he came near me. My mother did not know. He then made a pass at me when I was sixteen. When I refused him, he threw me out of the house.

AGB: Did you tell your mother then?

LM: It was a long and convoluted unfolding. The first time I left, when I was fifteen, what happened was this: he was yelling at my mother at the dining-room table. Her parents were visiting, and he was throwing a tantrum – very common for him – and I said, "You're such a bully! Why don't you stop picking on her?" And he picked up his plate and threw it at my head. I ducked and it hit an antique painting on the wall behind my head and broke it. He was furious, and tried to hurt me physically. My brother protected me – I mean, every one in the family was screaming at him to stop hitting me, but my brother was able to intervene enough for me to go into a room and shut a door and then run down the back staircase. Which is when I left. This is before the days of cellphones, so I was able to get to a payphone and call my boyfriend, who came and picked me up. I went to live with my dad, but did not get on well with my stepmother. Meanwhile, my brothers had both been thrown out of the house because my stepfather said: "Without Laura, there's no stepfamily left!" My mother kept begging me to come back, saying that things would be different, it would all be good, and … I went back. My reasons were complicated. I wanted to be near my boyfriend, I didn't get on with my stepmother, and my little brother, remember, was still there. So I went back, but within a short time, my stepfather made an aggressive pass at me, which I rebuffed, and he threw me out.

AGB: You have spoken about the pain behind rage; how anger is a mask for pain.

LM: When we feel something distressing, it doesn't feel good. So we try to … not feel it. Because feeling it puts us into a state of emergency, you know? This isn't just true for humans; it's true for all mammals. It's certainly true for dogs, who will bite if you drop something heavy on their paw. Pain causes us to lash out. We're protecting ourselves from danger. But what if it's just words, something that hurts our heart but not our body? We still lash out. It's an attempt to fend off the pain.

AGB: Don't you think that anger can also be constructive – for example, when establishing a boundary, making it clear that behaviour is unacceptable?

LM: Oh, absolutely. When I said pain, I should have been more specific. There are lots of different kinds of pain. We have grief – we get angry at the doctor who couldn't save the person we love; we have fear – we know that small dogs bark and growl more than big dogs because they're in fear more often. And we certainly know when our child does something wrong, we're scared that they're always going to be like that –

that they're never going to get potty trained or they're going to be an axe murderer or whatever – which is why we lash out. Powerlessness is a feeling we don't talk about so much. Feeling powerless is a terrible feeling; a life-threatening situation in some cases. Small animals, when upended, go into fight or flight and then freeze; they have a trauma response afterward. So powerlessness is a terrible feeling for us, and when we're establishing boundaries, it's often in response to that powerlessness, right?

AGB: Infringed on, yes.

LM: Again, that's hurt. We've been hurt. So it's absolutely an adaptive response to keeping someone from –

AGB: But it's not necessarily being hurt. Let me give you a military analogy. You cross the border. Crossing the border is inappropriate, a declaration of war. That's different from being hurt, isn't it? It's a recognition that someone is potentially dangerous, which is an entirely different thing.

LM: Well that's fear, then. Anger might be an appropriate response, but it's based on fear.

AGB: I think that anger, judiciously expressed, can be sanity. I've known lots of people who've taken their lives, and also lots of people who have capitulated to addiction, and so on. Without exception, not one of those people knew how to express anger to the people who had caused their suffering. They did not express their anger because they were taught that it is wrong to be angry. "Thou shalt honour thy father and thy mother" has been misinterpreted as meaning "thou shalt obey". My brother was the family diplomat; I was combative. And yet I was the only one who escaped.

LM: That's really interesting. Really interesting. Because in my family, I would say that I was more combative than either of my brothers, and I would say that I did better psychologically, so that's a very interesting point you're making.

AGB: You're an advocate of love, but when does your jaggedness emerge? Because you can't come from a background like yours and not have jaggedness.

LM: I think that in the beginning of my marriage, I took it out on my husband. I was thirty-one when I married, and had had a number of relationships. I think I was probably not a very good partner, you know? Because I just didn't know how to do it. I cheated on my first serious boyfriend, and so on. My father would say: "You're so smart and here you are sleeping with various guys and trying drugs. Why are you doing these things?" I had no idea why I was doing these things. It was hard for me to feel adequately loved by my husband. I would periodically have a tantrum – I would scream and yell. Luckily, my husband stayed calm during the tantrums –

AGB: A good man.

LM: A good man, yes. And at some point along the way, I realized that this was not who I wanted to be. Of course, I later drew on that experience to teach mothers to stop yelling.

AGB: You're talking about yelling, but I'm talking about an internal experience of jaggedness.

LM: In the beginning, I worked out my jaggedness by being highly competent and working very hard. I work harder than anybody I know, even my husband, and it's been the truth for most of my life. I worked very hard in college. I'm constantly trying to learn more, do better, work harder –

AGB: You run a private practice, are promoting a book, appear on television, do radio, run a demanding website, raise two children, and have a husband. Where do you find time for yourself?

LM: This has been my lifelong challenge. Even reading the books I want to read feels like I'm not being productive. Even just calling my friends! It's a challenge for me to stay connected to my friends, even the ones I love very much, because it feels like: "I've gotta get this email out! I've gotta answer this mothering letter!" As I'm not getting paid for most of it, I also have to make a living. I do meditate. There was a time before meditation when the issue behind slowing down was, for me, that there were tears waiting for me. I cried my way through meditation in the beginning.

AGB: But meditation is a formal relaxation; I'm talking about informal meditation. Exhaustion is endemic in the West, a critical problem, and inextricably connected with parenting problems because babies and children require our full emotional presence to blossom. Mothers so rarely talk to their babies any more in prams or strollers; they jog with the baby in tow, or listen to music on headphones, or text, as if the baby were no more than a dog to be walked. They don't take the opportunity to talk or sing to their babies, to introduce them to the world, to connect. I've seen the disconnection everywhere, most of it facilitated by technology. I've done it myself at times when I'm incredibly tired, rejecting my daughter in favour of staring at a screen. Which is why I refuse to buy a cellphone, or wear headphones, or own a radio, or use the television set for anything but DVDs and even then, only late at night. I mean, it's terrifying. Information is our currency, and yet so many of our children experience us as mute: staring, distracted, at machines, responsive only to technology. In part, this may be due to the fact that almost every mother I know is stressed out of her mind trying to keep up with the demands of work and family. What kind of life are we living?

LM: I agree with you. And in the United States in particular, our government policies are not just not family friendly, they're actually anti-family.

AGB: How is it possible to keep a family together when one or both parents are out twelve hours a day?

LM: It's very hard to keep a family together in those circumstances, which is why there are so many broken families. Unfortunately, what women are told is that children don't need them at home, and that in order to be whole people, women need to work outside the home. Don't get me wrong: I'm a feminist. The answer isn't to send women back into the kitchen. I certainly don't understand why as a culture, we think that children should be raised on the backs of women. The way to do it, I think, is to have both men and women share equally in child-rearing and in work outside the home. It's completely doable, but the corporate world doesn't really have a lot of interest in changing.

AGB: It's been shown that when monogamous primate

communities are established, parents begin to share care duties. This leads to the development of more complex brains as the infant is better protected and nurtured and its neural development isn't compromised by stress. When communities aren't monogamous, the males kill the offspring of other males so as to free their females for mating. So how do we go about loosening the corporate stranglehold on our lives so our males can increasingly share care duties? Because every child has a right to feel protected and free of stress.

LM: Well, the clinician Stanley Greenspan would have recommended the four-thirds solution. He said that if each parent stays at home with the child one third of the time and then works two thirds of the time, the child is home with the parents most of the time. And the child can be in care for the third third without it compromising the child's development. As a solution, I think that's not bad. There are lots of ways to do it, but Greenspan's suggestion alone would require that workplaces initiate jobsharing, benefits for part-time workers, and so on. We also need paid maternity and paternity leave, which we don't have in the States. All there is is six weeks through the healthcare side – that is, pregnancy is perceived as a health event that the woman is recovering from rather than respecting the postpartum period as necessary for a woman to bond with her baby. And it's only two-thirds of the pay, and it's for only six weeks, and it's only for some workers, and it's only for women, and it's only if you birth your baby, not if you adopt your baby. There are so many things that could be improved in government policy, and they would make an enormous difference.

AGB: So mothers need to assert their needs by making appointments to speak with their local politicians, and emailing or writing to their federal politicians?

LM: They do.

AGB: Now, you once described "that tough teen stage" as "completely unnecessary". It is created, you believe, by a parenting style that doesn't meet the needs of adolescents.

LM: Parents forget what it's like to be a teenager. Most parents, when their teenagers yell at them, yell back. If they only took a deep breath instead, said, "I'm sorry, sweetie, that things are so hard at the moment". More often than not, your children will cry when you show empathy. Because that's what they needed to do in the first place: cry. And then, after a good cry, they can talk about the stresses in their lives, because the stresses on teenagers today are huge.

AGB: What I've observed is that a lot of parents punish and/or ostracize their children when the child's behaviour reveals the fractures and elisions within the family.

LM: Of course, this totally destroys the relationship.

AGB: I've known some terrifyingly inept mothers, but you're not allowed to say this as there's a kind of conspiratorial silence around motherhood: however bad the mother, it is perceived as bad form to point it out, no matter how deeply the children are suffering. We all have to suspend judgment. And yet children are judged without mercy. I think that as a community, we need to stop blaming children and see them for what they are: as mirrors of our own capacity to love.

LM: A lot of parents have trouble taking responsibility for their actions because it is such a terrible thing to have done. Being given a child to raise is such a sacred responsibility. How can a parent come to peace with themselves when they've hurt their child? Most of the time, parents don't do what you did: you found yourself spanking your child and couldn't believe it, so you went and got help in order to stop. But most parents who spank their children tell themselves that it was necessary; they tell themselves that the child required the spanking, that it helped the child's behaviour. Despite the fact that all the research we have shows that it never helps behaviour.

AGB: I never thought that it helped Bethesda. In retrospect, all it did was help me release aggression and stress in the short-term; in the long-term, I felt like I wanted to die of shame. Our needs were clashing; she wasn't conforming when I needed her to. Through her behaviour, she was telling me that she was stressed and frightened and needed my tenderness and attention; through my behaviour, I was telling her that I had no tenderness or affection left to give – I was running on empty; I needed tenderness and affection, but none was available.

LM: Parents blame and punish their children because then they don't feel like bad people. And they do the same with their teenagers. They can't believe that they've created such a monster, right?

AGB: Laura, what is the solution? Does the mothering community have to open a dialogue about frailty? Because all we seem to be open about are the secondary emotions – the rage, the depression – rather than core feelings of pain and vulnerability.

LM: Such a great question, and such a complicated question. I would say, first of all, that expressing feelings in words means that you don't have to act on those feelings. To shame mothers about their aggressive feelings for their own children would not have the desired effect; to do so would only make them put their sadistic feelings in the closet and take it out on their children in private. However, I think there's a big range in being verbal. Being verbal in the privacy of a therapist's office is one thing, but it's totally another to do it online. These days, we live online. Our lives are so public that we're no longer sure what should be public and what should be private. Which is why I set a rule: if it's something that would disturb our child to hear, whatever their age, we shouldn't be saying it in public. And I really don't think it's appropriate for mothers to be talking in detail in public about wanting to hurt their children, because I think that their children will one day discover that, and I can't even imagine how wounding that would be for the child.

AGB: The issue of a child's right to privacy, to dignity – that has to be paramount.

LM: Right.

AGB: So how can we be more supportive of our children?

LM: We can make a real effort to see things from their point of view. Often when I tell parents to empathize, they say, "I told my son he was angry, and he got even angrier!" And I reply, "That's because you didn't empathize – you analysed and labelled." But if we didn't get a lot of empathy ourselves growing up, we're confused by what empathy means, you know? Empathy literally means to feel from someone else's perspective. The golden rule is really to treat others as we would like to be treated, which means understanding that children have a reason for what they're doing. It may not be a good reason, but they do have a reason. Parents need to practise compassion.

AGB: How can we better show our children that we love them?

LM: Well, the most important is physical touch. I'm a great believer in the old adage: twelve hugs a day for growth! There's nothing more effective than a five-minute cuddle when you wake up in the morning with each child. If you have four children, that can take twenty minutes, but it'll make your whole morning go so much more easily. All it takes is a cuddle every morning to reconnect, because kids experience sleep like going to Siberia. When we reconnect in the morning, it helps them regain the desire to co-operate with us, and then when we're reunited later in the day – presuming you've been apart during the day for whatever period of time – a snuggle and cuddle really makes a huge difference. Roughhousing is also a great idea. You want to get your children giggling. Roughhousing helps them release anxieties they've built up in the course of their day. As I said, all small humans have fears, and anxiety is just another word for fear. All children walk back into our homes with some build-up of anxiety, of fear. And if they get a chance to laugh, it's nature's way of releasing that anxiety and fear, so that anxiety and fear don't determine their behaviour.

AGB: I've always believed in the necessity of encouragement.

LM: Encouragement is necessary to keep our spirits up and do hard things because life is full of hard things. I mean, just think about the age-appropriate things every child is asked to do on a regular basis – start a new school, start with a new teacher, figure out where the bathroom is in the new school, make a new friend, tie shoelaces, ride a bike, read! These all take some gumption. So of course kids need our encouragement. Children are designed to take chances and explore and grow, but the only way they can grow so quickly, learn so much and take so many risks is when we're there as back-up. Only when they know we're there – when we give them the encouragement to keep trying even though something may be hard – can they find the spirit to keep trying. It's hard to imagine a child really thriving and reaching their full potential without someone backing them.

AGB: Do you think that as a culture, we have forgotten that childhood is not just a series of developmental stages? Have we forgotten the garden of dreams that childhood is at its best?

LM: Yes, I totally do. Oh, my goodness! Children are joy-filled, they are exuberant, they are fully alive; they haven't damped down their aliveness and their creativity the way that most of us, as adults, have learned to do. And so if we are in the moment playing with our children, we can relearn how to play. Most mothers tell me, "I don't wanna play with my kids! I hate to play!" But the truth is, play is good for us, too. We don't do it because we're trying to ram our kids through these schedules of homework and bathtime and bedtime, and we forget that that's not life, that's just a schedule, and to be fully alive children actually need us to participate with them in life in a way that's not just about schedules. When we're really there in the moment and spontaneously playing, anything could arise, anything could happen. Because that's what that creativity is: possibility.

AGB: There are moments with my daughter that make me feel as close to God – or whatever we understand as God – as it is possible to be. I remember when she was a big baby, maybe eight months old, we'd get up at some unholy hour around dawn to breastfeed, and I would sit with her in my lap in the kitchen, her head on my breast and with my arms around her, just rocking this warm baby in my lap as the sun rose. The sense of spiritual fusion was irreplaceable; I mean, it was just complete happiness.

LM: I remember my son as a toddler in the garden, digging and finding worms. I remember his joy not only in discovering the natural world, but that he could wield a shovel. And I remember him looking at me with such love as a toddler. Nobody had ever looked at me with that kind of love before. I was almost embarrassed in front of his gaze, because I didn't see how I could be worthy of such unmitigated adoration. And I felt the exact same thing with my daughter. I feel lucky beyond belief to be their mother; I love these two people more than I could ever express. In a garden, you see a flower blossom once and it's gone; but children blossom over and over and over again, constantly growing and changing, becoming more themselves all the time. So you see them more deeply as they get older. I just feel so lucky to be able to have been their witness.

Laura Markham's guide to joyful parenting

1. Regulate your own emotions.
2. Be your child's advocate and don't give up on her.
3. Punishment always worsens your child's behaviour. Instead, set limits on behaviour while empathizing with feelings.
4. Kids need a safe place to express feelings while you listen. If you want to raise a child who can manage his behaviour, he first has to manage the emotions that drive that behaviour. And if you want a child who can manage his emotions, he first needs to know he has a safe place (your arms) to cry and rage where he won't be shushed.
5. Remember: she's just a kid, trying as hard as she can. Expect age-appropriate behaviour, not perfection, and keep your priorities straight.
6. Don't take it personally. Whatever your child does, it will be a lot easier for you to respond peacefully if you notice when you start getting triggered.
7. All misbehaviour comes from basic needs that aren't met.
8. The best parenting expert is your child. Let him show you what he needs, from infancy on. Listen with your heart. Be willing to change and grow – and learn to enjoy the process.
9. What worked yesterday may not work tomorrow, so your parenting approach needs to evolve as your kids do.
10. Stay connected and never withdraw your love, even for a moment. Above all, safeguard your relationship with your child.

ahaparenting.com

The emotional impact of IVF

The price of yearning

All his friends were having kids,
and he wanted to have kids so badly.

In 1978, Louise Brown, the first in-vitro fertilization (IVF) baby, was born in Manchester, England; since then, over three million have been born around the world. The numbers are significant. Over 30,000 women undergo IVF treatment each year in the UK alone, and 10,000 babies result. It is predicted that in a quarter of a century – and partly because of the established global trend for delayed motherhood – one in three births will involve IVF. In response, Nichola Bedos, the widely published psychotherapist and infant mental health specialist, has written *IVF and Ever After: The Emotional Needs of Families*, a compassionate and deeply insightful examination of, and guide through, the intense emotional impact of IVF on parents and their "miracle" children.

In global terms, the tally is disturbing. Some 80 million people are infertile. And for those considering treatment, skilled psychological support is critical: emotional complexities must be explored before IVF can be attempted. Bedos observes: "Arriving at the door of an infertility clinic without having reflected on the feelings evoked by a diagnosis of infertility can be disastrous."

The aftermath of successful and unsuccessful IVF cycles not only affects the immediate family, but a wider circle of relatives and, ultimately, the community at large. Because of the increasingly effective technology, infertile and older couples, carriers of genetic abnormalities and same-sex couples can now become biological families. The problem?

Funnelled through prejudice, IVF has the potential to hurt humanity itself. "If IVF could produce the gender requested by parents for cultural reasons, it could also lead to serious shifts in the make-up of a society", Bedos writes. "In this instance, we [would be] able to achieve scientific change that may not necessarily benefit us as a species."

IVF, she reminds us, presents challenges on almost every level, particularly the ethical.

"First", Bedos says, "the world needs to decide the fate of the six million frozen embryos that exist, and how we can meet the emotional needs of the parents of these embryos while also as professionals, witnessing the pain of couples whose own embryos fail to implant. Second, we have the needs and rights of unborn children to consider as we try to decide whether surrogacy is permitted, whether same-sex couples have equal access to treatment and whether single women are able to undergo treatment. And third, we have the issue over the size of the fertility business and whether the large income stream generated by the treatment all over the world also facilitates the provision of unbiased and fair advice for couples who come to clinics seeking advice."

And then there are medico-legal questions and religious, emotional and physical questions, both for parents and their children, who may later contend with issues about their genetic heritage and sense of identity. These issues are anything but minor. The incidence of certain birth defects has been discovered to be tenfold in IVF babies. Storing fertilized embryos can trigger genetic changes causing mental disorders in later life. The fertility of babies can be severely compromised by IVF drugs. Last year, the Australian Institute for Health and Welfare found that the IVF baby death rate is twice that of the naturally conceived: one in fifty is stillborn or dies within a month of birth. And there are greater risks of early labour, premature birth, lower birthweight and chronic conditions such as cerebral palsy. The impact of stress on IVF couples, too, cannot be discounted.

Research has demonstrated that elevated stress hormone levels interfere with fertility levels in both women and men. Acupuncture has been shown to increase the likelihood of IVF success, although accurate research data is not currently available to pinpoint the exact mechanism; it is believed that acupuncture treatment reduces the levels of diagnosis- or treatment-triggered stress hormones circulating in the woman's body. But the journey remains arduous for many and, in the end, impossible for some. The drop-out rate – estimated to be over 60 per cent – is attributed to anxiety and grief.

When Michelle Fragias, thirty-one, and her husband first discovered she was pregnant with triplets during her second IVF cycle, they were elated. "Most days even now I can't even go there", she explains. "That pregnancy was a rollercoaster. One of the identical twins had a very rare disease called the Pentalogy of Cantrell, so there was a chance she'd die or that all of them would. We were advised to terminate the pregnancy, at nineteen weeks" – her voice grows unsteady – "I went into labour, had the contractions and delivered three girls. As I said, I just can't go there some days." She begins to weep. "It's just too hard. My twin boys were born during the third cycle. They keep me going."

Over four cycles, Leigh Buntine, thirty-six, gave birth to two sets of twins. "We lost one of the first set to a neural tube defect", she says. "Tyson was born alive and died ten minutes later. The neural tube defect was discovered at our twelve-week ultrasound. The condition is anencephaly, which means that the skull doesn't form properly. It's usually attributed to lack of folate, but I took folate."

She pauses. "There was just a lot of grief, really. We were told that there was a severe risk to Riley, the healthy twin – had Tyson died in utero, Riley would have been at severe risk. It was very hard to cope with the anxiety. I was a mess. If I didn't feel them move for half an hour, I'd panic. The time in between doctor visits was just awful. I'd sit down and reflect, holding my tummy and thinking: this is the only time I'm going to be able to hold my two boys."

Between the birth of each set of twins, Buntine developed breast cancer. "I had a mastectomy", she quietly says. "Six months of chemotherapy, and eight months later I was told I could have IVF. I was lucky; I had embryos in storage. They would otherwise have denied me another cycle. But I feel the cancer was caused by the fertility drugs. I think there is a direct relationship, but of course you can't say that."

Bedos is careful. "My concerns with IVF treatment lie with the fact that as a relatively new technique, we have little data to show any long-term patterns", she says.

Women who pursue the process are saddled with such unnerving possibilities. Clots, ovarian hyperstimulation syndrome and cancers are all possible outcomes. Parents undergoing IVF are also nine times more likely to produce twins than non-IVF parents.

Over 50 per cent of women using IVF also struggle to care for their newborns after c-sections. More than half of all IVF mothers switch to bottle-feeding in the first three months, citing failure to establish a "good" milk supply. And IVF parents experience that which Bedos calls "a pervasive fear of loss" kindled before the IVF treatment process. Bedos believes that as a result of these and other factors, IVF can significantly complicate both the parental relationship and the experience of parenthood. The unfulfilled wish for a baby – which Bedos describes as "felt keenly by both sexes" – is traumatic in itself. "A woman feels an intense longing that covers everything in life with a deep sense of sadness", she says, "whereas men often experience an unfulfilled wish to reproduce as anxiety; they work very hard, become withdrawn and feel less confident."

Dr Bruce Perry, a leading American trauma specialist, has spearheaded research into how children's brains work and how they are affected by trauma. It is now known that the brain of an unborn baby whose mother suffers a highly traumatic experience will be bathed in stress hormones that will permanently change it. The unparalleled sensitivity of babies to life experiences from conception onwards clearly indicates that families must be helped to create the best possible environment for their children, if only for the benefit of the community. Couples traumatized by IVF also benefit from caring professional assistance to help alleviate some of the damage.

Bedos explains how gender determines the way in which we deal with stress. "The wiring of the male and female brain is actually very different. Women tend to ask for support, talk things over, cry and show signs that they are in need of help. Men withdraw; they may throw themselves into work and become distant. These reactions, if not understood, can cause a lot of hurt. The best exercise I teach couples is to listen but not try to fix anything. Men, particularly, hate to see their partners distressed and will try to make things better, but women rarely see this as helpful."

Leigh Buntine is quiet for a moment. "I'd felt like I'd failed because everyone knew it was me who had the problem", she acknowledges. "We were always quick to point out – to preserve my husband's sense of masculinity – that it wasn't him. Infertility really impacted my sense of femininity. The doctor said that with polycystic syndrome there was a chance I would grow a moustache and hairs on my chest. And I guess that I felt guilty that Andrew married me and I couldn't give him children. All his friends were having kids, and he wanted to have kids so badly. Trying all the time took the fun out of it. We'd always talked about having kids, and I felt like I'd failed him. I guess I felt less of a woman than my girlfriends. It really takes something away from you. Little girls play with dolls. That's what girls do; they grow up and have babies."

In addition, the physical, emotional and financial demands of IVF can rapidly erode parental optimism. "The transition to parenthood poses unexpected challenges", Bedos says. "Anxiety about the ability to sustain the baby, a loss of confidence regarding the capacity to care for the baby, and feeding and settling difficulties. Successful maternal–infant bonding requires that the mother be emotionally available for her child. By this I mean that a mum is focused on her baby, can accept the emotions that come with early mothering – vulnerability, fear of not being good enough – and can also cope with the baby's feelings of despair when tired, hungry and overstimulated."

Mothers who are overly stressed, depressed or traumatized have to utilize most of their energy to manage their own emotions, meaning they are less able to focus on their babies. The babies, feeling this lack of responsiveness, withdraw into themselves, resulting in what Bedos calls "improper attachment" and an anxious baby.

Numerous issues faced by IVF couples are similar to those confronted by adoptive parents – namely, a sense of failure to conceive naturally, the emotionally turbulent process of having a child, and fears over bonding. The one issue that

Bedos believes sets IVF couples apart is that repeated – and common – IVF failures become personalized.

"I wouldn't say that anger is a huge problem with IVF families, but irritability certainly is", she says. "Stressful and traumatic experiences lead to nervous system arousal as the body gears up to meet an intense challenge, and when that challenge continues for months, even years, it leaves the body permanently ready to fight or run away from danger. Couples who suffer this nervous system arousal will find arguments are very frequent and can be hard to end. They become angry and depressed with themselves, which sharply lowers their self-esteem. In contrast, difficulties with adoption give parents external forces to blame – the agency, DOCS, foreign protocol, and so on."

And then, of course, there is the procedure itself, which is frequently experienced as disruptive by women. High hormonal dosages and extreme performance anxiety result in emotional instability, leaving male partners to feel doubly impotent. "Men often leave the emotions about pregnancy, birth and early parenting to women, feeling that male culture does not warrant emotion and that the women's emotions are often so big anyway there is no room for their emotions too", Bedos says.

Having witnessed the worst effects of IVF, Bedos understands how dehumanizing technological interference can be, corroding the relationships of couples and those between mothers and newborns; these babies, their mothers feel, aren't their own. The ability to test for and diagnose many fertility issues has had a positive impact in that treatment can be offered, but it also makes diagnosed partners feel devalued, as though they had deliberately caused the issue, and these feelings can be very destructive.

"We're instinctively primed to view baby-making as the byproduct or aim of an established, loving relationship", Bedos says. "Our survival as a species depends on men and women forging close relationships to provide the care that dependent children need. Such instincts ensure that love and romance are significant components of conception. And IVF can interrupt this normal love-protection-procreation pathway, as strangers take control over a moment designed solely for two lovers.

IVF couples don't even get to choose the date of conception, never mind the time or location!"

Privacy in particular is important in matters of conception for both men and women. In the case of a woman, the urge to conceive is accompanied by a withdrawal into herself, a need to summon the energy and belief to create life. Invasive medical tests rupture this internalization and create a disconnection between a woman and her body.

Michelle Fragias and her husband abstained from sex after conception, fearing "the embryo would be hurt by the sperm", but Buntine simply found the procedure intrusive. "Instead of living the fairytale, we handed over the romance to the doctors at the clinic", she says.

Such depersonalization can lead to difficulties in the early days of motherhood, as described earlier. Buntine didn't experience that fabled "rush of love" when her first set of twins were born. "They were taken away from me", she says flatly. "I didn't see them for two days because I was recovering from the caesarean. Riley was born at thirty-two weeks and was in intensive care for five weeks, and I didn't fall in love with him until he was eight weeks old. I liked him and knew I should love him, but I didn't have that immediate I-would-do-anything-for-this-child sort of love. The birth was all just so clinical. It was like it was happening to someone else. I'd had these children, but they didn't feel mine. I could see them, but I couldn't take them away. Riley's twin, Tyson, died during his Apgar test. Why they bothered, I'll never know, as they knew he would die."

Her pause is heartbreaking. "We never even heard him cry."

Identity, too, is rarely considered. Around 30 per cent of parents interviewed after egg, sperm or embryo donation claimed they intended to withhold the fact from their children. Information about the child's origins is stifled for fear that he will seek a relationship with the biological parent, and that this relationship could then usurp their own.

"Identity is formed even before the baby is born, through the baby's experiences", Bedos explains. "Babies who are nurtured, handled gently, and who have most of their needs met promptly grow up to have a healthy sense of being good, deserving love and of being ultimately useful members of society. Truthful information about how a child came to be is crucial to all children. Secrecy about a child's origins is toxic because withholding information about a child's origins leads to him developing a false sense of identity. When he discovers the truth, his view of himself is shattered and he loses all trust in his parents. From the beginning, these children need to be told in very simple terms that they were adopted, came from a donor or were conceived in a special way."

At every turn, Bedos demonstrates the value of counselling before, during and after the IVF procedure. Preventative counselling can, she insists, reduce the impact and longevity of trauma. Counselling also helps previously traumatized people process stifled emotions lest they compound the intensity of the new traumatic experience.

"Couples who have counselling before treatment are more realistic about the process", Bedos says. "This means that they have a better idea of what to expect, and can cope with the emotional highs and lows more positively. They are also able to articulate their feelings to each other, producing much greater teamwork. IVF parents need plenty of reassurance that they are doing a fantastic job – and they generally are!"

Fragias describes her husband as profoundly supportive, but the marriage was strained by the loss of their triplets. "He fell into a depression", she says. "We tried to see a counsellor, but no-one can understand what you've been through unless you've been there. I threw myself into work – the only way I could get through the day was by working long hours. I didn't understand what was wrong with my husband. We just weren't intimate. In the end, he had to do something for himself, so he gave up smoking, and to this day he hasn't picked up a cigarette. I've been told I haven't grieved properly, but I guess people handle it in different ways. It's a part of me now, and I accept that. Every year, we let off three balloons on the day they died. My boys will do that, too."

Bedos urges couples considering IVF to visit at least one clinic for an exploratory discussion, and to seek second opinions if they feel uncertain. She also recommends temporarily eliminating unnecessary obligations to friends and family. Couples undergoing treatment need "pleasant time" – dinner, a walk, watching a movie, privacy. And once they become parents, they "need to understand the stress they have been through and to adjust the expectations they have of themselves. I always help IVF parents think of times they can just 'be' with their babies or children; not teaching them anything, worrying if they are unwell or feeling the need to be very close, simply lying on a picnic rug on a sunny day chatting to a baby or lying on the sofa together enjoying a funny movie. These moments are to be treasured as a reward for the stress of conception."

As a race, Bedos notes, we are not very good at sensing emotional crises. "Ancient cultures used to spend time fire-gazing and interacting extensively with others", she laughs, "meaning they had time to reflect and talk about feelings. Our way of life ensures that we have little time for reflection on how we're feeling and how our lives are unfolding, and even less time to talk about it. Consequently, emotional crises rear up seemingly out of nowhere. I ask [IVF parents] to listen to their partners for five minutes a night without doing anything more than holding hands and saying 'I'm here,' and then to reflect on what was said."

In the end, Buntine adores her three children, and Fragias agrees that the expense and trauma were worth it. "I'd do it all again in a heartbeat!" she exclaims. "How else could I have had my beautiful boys? They've made my life complete."

Nichola Bedos's guide to peace for IVF parents

1. Each parent needs to find someone they can confide in. IVF and parenting after IVF can bring up large and sometimes unexpected feelings, which is why a confidante is helpful.

2. Find regular time to be out of the house and away from the kids to talk, swap experiences and keep in touch with each other.

3. Find a really good GP you trust and feel comfortable with. Going through IVF can increase stress and anxiety, and a reassuring GP for parents and baby alike makes a huge difference.

4. Have a stress management plan – each parent will benefit from adopting a few techniques used regularly such as regular gym visits, an exercise class, a shopping trip, yoga or meditation.

5. Try to keep parenting expectations realistic. Stress and anxiety can often make you expect too much of yourself. If you feel you aren't doing a good job, talk it over with someone you trust.

6. Aim for a spontaneous family fun day out once a month where you let go of time, expectations and the busyness of everyday life and simply enjoy being mum or dad.

7. Don't hope that relationship conflict will "go away". If you're arguing more than you'd like, seek relationship counselling. Thriving as a family after IVF often requires some professional input.

8. Be upfront with your child about his or her origins once they're old enough to understand.

9. Smile whenever you can. Enjoy the little moments – that first smile, the cuddles, the first words mispronounced. Try not to be so stressed that these moments of joy pass you by.

10. Don't be afraid to ask for help. Many IVF parents can feel so blessed with their longed-for baby that they become unwilling or unable to stop pretending all is well and they can do it alone. Remember: it takes a whole community to raise a child.

facebook.com/nsbedos

The legacy of purpose

A conversation with Stephanie Coontz

There aren't enough hours in the day for any woman or man to be a great career person, a great partner and a great parent.

On stage, Stephanie Coontz – confident, diminutive and with an ironic penchant for clerical purple – is a dazzling speaker. Arguably the world's foremost family historian, she's at her best with those with whom she disagrees, rolling her big kohled eyes at their faux pas, crossing those slim black-stockinged legs and levelling opponents with a slew of statistics. Her contribution to the debate about women's rights and the maternal paradigm is invaluable. Coontz has always riled against the imposition of absolutes, barracking for parity even when parity can be construed as an absolute in itself. It's a show and no mistaking it, but her credentials are real. She has testified about her research before the House Select Committee on Children, Youth and Families in Washington, DC, and lectured all over the world. Her bestselling books include *A Strange Stirring: The Feminine Mystique and American Women at the Dawn of the 1960s; Marriage, a History: How Love Conquered Marriage; The Way We Really Are: Coming to Terms with America's Changing Families* and *The Way We Never Were: American Families and the Nostalgia Trap*, and her byline is familiar to readers of *The New York Times, The Wall Street Journal* and *Vogue*. Currently a faculty member at Washington's Evergreen State College, Coontz, who turns seventy-one this year, is Director of Research and Public Education for the Council on Contemporary Families. Privately, she is both saltier and more vulnerable than her public swagger would suggest.

AGB: So how exactly is a Stephanie Coontz created?

SC: My mother was, off and on, a housewife, and then a ship-fitter at the Seattle docks during the Second World War, and then a housewife again, and then an English teacher. My father went back to school on the GI bill after being a merchant marine, and then he was a union organizer, and then he became a professor of economics.

AGB: What did you learn through observing your mother? Was she a frustrated housewife?

SC: When I was about six or seven, she used to take those Gallo wine jugs and paint pretty pictures on them, and I remember thinking, 'Oh, how artistic my mother is!' Years later, she told me that story as a sign of just how desperately bored and unhappy she was.

AGB: You didn't perceive that she was bored and unhappy?

SC: She faked it very well for us girls! [laughs]

AGB: My mother longed for a life outside the house.

SC: A lot of people of that generation told me that it was only after reading *The Feminine Mystique* that they came to understand their mothers' anger and irritability.

AGB: My brother and I were very aware of our mother's depression and frustration. Everything she did was done with resentment – cooking, childcare, housework. The opposite was the case with my grandmothers, who both worked all their lives.

SC: That certainly ties in with all the research. We do know now that women who work all their lives tend to be happier and healthier at age forty and less subject to depression.

AGB: Do you think those results may be skewed by the fact that we live in a culture in which mothering has been devalued? Of course a stay-at-home mother is going to feel depressed and frustrated in a culture in which mothering is understood as a menial task.

SC: Some people think that mothers are unhappy today because society doesn't value their contributions the way it used to, but wherever motherhood has been romanticized it has also been used to deny the individual personhood of women. Throughout most of the twentieth century, the sentimentalization of the mother co-existed with a vicious hostility toward mothers who actually tried to exercise their supposed influence in the home. Even in the nineteenth century, before boys were teased and bullied if they expressed love for their mother, many women were made desperately unhappy by their imprisonment in a one-sided identity that forced them to deny any other desires or inclinations.

AGB: But was the nature of motherhood responsible for their desperate unhappiness, or did motherhood take the fall for other factors, such as the way women were treated by men and the culture in general?

SC: I think that you're probably right; those factors would skew the results.

AGB: What expectations did you have of marriage and motherhood?

SC: I just expected it. That's what you grew up with in the 1950s and 1960s. Here is my fantasy when I was in college: "Gosh, I'd like to marry a man who would be willing to build me a separate part of the house for my study." It never occurred to me that I could build it myself! I wanted to marry a man who would build me "a room of one's own", you know? And before college, I wanted to fight the Nazis. I was a romantic; I wanted to go to Spain and gallop across the plains fighting Franco with Yul Brynner at my side! [laughs] So I loved school, I had romantic fantasies, and men and marriage were involved.

AGB: Do you think that's a bad thing?

SC: [pauses] My generation of women grew up expecting too much from marriage. I remember that when I dated a boy in high school, I would write down my first name against his last name to see how it would look. I think it's a lot healthier when women are brought up to think of marriage as something great if it happens, but if it doesn't happen, that's fine too.

AGB: What are the most important lessons you've learned regarding marriage?

SC: My own? The less you need it, either economically or emotionally, the more you can give to it. I am married to my college sweetheart but in between we broke up and I made an error, and ended up a single mother for many years. I don't talk about how that error came about because it's not something I want to burden my son with, or make him feel bad about. So.

AGB: What happens when baby comes along and there's no marriage?

SC: That's the big conundrum. For better-educated, more economically secure couples, those babies cannot come along, either because they use contraception willingly or because they resort to abortion. But for many less-educated and lower-income couples, the majority of conceptions are, as my colleague Paula England put it, not quite accidental, not quite planned. It's hard for people to defer gratification indefinitely, and they think: "Well, maybe we'll just roll the dice and see what happens. And if it happens, it's meant to be." If a child then comes along, social conservatives believe that the couple should marry, but the evidence on that is very mixed. Kids whose parents marry after the birth do not do better – and, in some cases, do worse – than kids who are born to a stable, unwed mother who remains unwed and doesn't go through what sociologist Andrew Cherlin calls the "churning" situation of having many partners move in and out. I would certainly say to anyone I know, "DO NOT GET PREGNANT UNTIL YOU'RE READY TO HAVE A SUPPORTIVE PARTNER WITH YOU!" But it's one thing for me to say that to my son or to your daughter, and another to say it to someone who lives in a neighbourhood where even the few people who graduate from high school are functionally illiterate, where there are no jobs on the horizon, and where there are very few models of people who have deferred gratification and ended up with a good life rather than being shot or ending up alone. It's just so tempting in those circumstances for people to think: "Hell, why shouldn't I bring a child up in the world? At least it will bring me some happiness!"

AGB: In the West, the devaluing of love has resulted in a trivialization of motherhood. Women are bamboozled into believing that motherhood is only one priority among many and easily managed, rather than having it realistically presented as a revolution. Mothering a child involves an unparalleled emotional, energetic and spiritual expenditure.

SC: There aren't enough hours in the day for any woman or man to be a great career person, as well as a great partner and also a great parent.

AGB: Interestingly, male politicians are never criticized for being absent from their families and/or inept fathers; such issues are never raised.

SC: For me, it's not the devaluation of motherhood that is bothersome, but the devaluation of caregiving. If you don't value caregiving at all levels to all people, then no matter how much you romanticize it, it becomes trivialized and it becomes much more difficult to carry off.

AGB: But motherhood is the very matrix of value; that is where we learn to value caregiving. You've written extensively about the romanticizing of motherhood – Erica Jong called it 'an orgy of motherphilia' – but I have found the opposite to be true; women are now bombarded with the romanticizing of career and conditioned to understand paid work as superior in every way to the experience of mothering a child, where, in fact, the average job is tedious, underpaid and stressful.

SC: I agree with you that careers are romanticized, but motherhood is sentimentalized.

AGB: But careers are, too.

SC: No, I don't think the language is the same.

AGB: Middle-class girls in particular have careers presented to them with the same level of hyperbole with which the Victorians addressed motherhood. Let me give you an example. Ignoring the fact that the majority of female workers are concentrated in poorly remunerated and physically demanding occupations such as retailing, cleaning and clerical work ("Working Girls" by Alison Wolf, *Prospect*, April 2006), author Gail Sheehy presented paid employment to women as offering the same spiritual renewal attributed by priests to religious conversion:

"If women had wives to keep house for them, to stay home with vomiting children, get the car fixed, fight with the painters, run to the supermarket, reconcile the bank statements, listen to everyone's problems, cater the dinner parties, and nourish the spirit each night, just imagine the possibilities for expansion – the number of books that would be written, companies started, professorships filled, political offices that would be held, by women." (*Passages: Predictable Crises of Adult Life*, EP Dutton, 1976, p. 157) Here Sheehy is not, of course, addressing all women, for if women of the developing world were also writing books, starting companies, and so on, who would stay home with the vomiting children of First World mothers? Sheehy's use of language must also be noted. In association with childcare: "vomiting", "broken", "fight", "run" and "problems"; in association with career, "imagine", "possibilities", "expansion", "books", "filled" and "held".

SC: I firmly believe that women, like men, need a balance between work and career and caregiving. I do think it's important not to forget that even work that seems boring to us can give people a sense of satisfaction, and there are a lot of psychological studies showing that. If it's not really high urgency, high demand and totally inflexible, even fairly boring work, such as serving food, involves interaction with someone other than a child. And that's important to women.

AGB: In the UK, a significant proportion of working mothers have said that they would prefer to stay home with their young children, but that they're being screwed by the economy.

SC: I'm very leery of those polls, because most of them come down to mood. If you really word them carefully, most women and men would like fewer working hours – a thirty-hour working week, which would give them time to do other things.

AGB: Thirty hours is a delicious fantasy. You've written that as of 2000, the average working couple works a combined 82-hour working week, while almost 15 per cent of married couples had a joint working week of 100 hours or more. Is this just me, or does this seem completely insane to you?

SC: It's insane! It's absolutely insane, particularly in countries – and it's not just America – where worker productivity has expanded immensely and workers have got nothing from it. Their real wages have stagnated, and they don't even get time off. It's ridiculous!

AGB: The solution?

SC: It seems perfectly obvious to me that we have not only the technological skills and capacity to produce the things we need with far fewer working hours per week, but that we experience a real social benefit from doing so – freeing up the overworked to spend time enjoying life and taking care of family, and freeing up the underworked, so that they're not miserably poor.

AGB: What are the repercussions of these insane hours on relationships?

SC: I think that they're worse on marriages than they are on kids. What we've found is that women cut back on activities like shopping and housecleaning and try to make extra time with their kids, but one of the ways they do that is by multitasking. Women do a lot of subdividing – "Here, you take this kid and go to soccer; I'll take that kid and go shopping." This is how the couple loses one of the most important things for couples, which is time without the kids. One of the most persistent, effective predictors of happiness for couples is spending social time with other adults. And that is what couples who work these insane hours yet try to be fair to their kids give up.

AGB: It's such a bind. There are only twenty-four hours in a day.

SC: But they're giving up their social time, which is so important to marital satisfaction. If you go out with other people, you get a chance to show off your partner, hear new jokes and learn new information, which really is a shot in the arm for a marriage.

AGB: It's not even a matter of time constraints, it's a matter of energy. Couples are exhausted. It's not about running out of conversation, but being too tired to have a conversation. I know couples who literally sit, fogged, in front of the television every night until bedtime. The fag-end of a day isn't quality time for anyone. Two adults come home after a long day – exhausted, depleted – and have to summon playfulness for a child who has been yearning for them since breakfast. These children very quickly learn that intimacy is not the priority.

SC: From my perspective, the same things that have taught us to want more depth, more intimacy and more equality are also part and parcel of other things. The social and economic changes that have increased interpersonal equality and intimacy have also increased careerism, competitive pressure, and this increasingly frenetic work life. So instead of saying we've lost the intimacy, it's that we can't have the intimacy we want unless we somehow find a better balance.

AGB: In this vein, you've often referred to a "caregiving crisis". Has this always been the case?

SC: One reason there wasn't so much of a crisis before was due to the high death rates; you didn't have ageing parents to take care of at the same time you had kids. Also, if you want to go back to medieval times, there were great class differences. But now we live in a society that has – admirably – the idea that everybody deserves care; that there should not be any child labour; that old people shouldn't be put on an ice-floe and sent off to die –

AGB: Although in some cases, that wouldn't be such a bad idea –

SC: [laughing] We now have a greater need for caregiving because kids aren't sent out to work at an early age and lifespans are lengthened, but even though we have these values, we've done nothing to put them in practice. We've made caregiving, once again, something that has to be done by women, and something that does not get any kind of social support.

AGB: But women are hormonally primed to look after infants in a way that men are not. When a baby is born, what Michel Odent calls "a cocktail of love hormones" is released in women. Not to mention breastfeeding. Men are simply not biologically equipped the same way.

SC: Whatever the differences between women and men, we now organize work and our social and economic lives in ways that tell us that caregiving should be democratic, but we have no social institutions to help people act upon these new values and to spread them around fairly.

AGB: I've also observed a chronological apartheid, where you have children put in care and then school – the institutionalization of childhood – and adults working themselves into cardiac arrests alongside their coevals, while the old are stored in aged-care facilities until their expiry dates are up. What is lost in the wash is love. There is a world of difference between the experience of "care" – the wiping of a bottom, the bathing of a body: basic biological obligations – and intimacy.

SC: I share the indignation that this exists at all, but caution against the painting of too negative a picture –

AGB: A 2006 World Health Organization report stated that almost a million people commit suicide each year, outranking homicides or the casualties of war; global suicide rates have increased by 60 per cent over the past forty-five years. Rates of antidepressant use are skyrocketing, as are sleeping pill prescriptions. Our jails are overflowing. The decrease in human happiness is marked, and dovetails with changes in both the time we spend with those we love and the way we parent our children.

SC: I don't know the international rates of suicide, but there are several factors in the creation of the new nuclear family isolation. One is the way housing and transportation have evolved, with people moving to suburbs and chasing better homes and schools. The way that we've constructed shopping, travel and work has made it necessary for families to separate and strike out on their own. And with the rising age of marriage, we're seeing so many young people understand that they have to develop their own network of friends, you know? They can't just go, like people in the 1950s and 1960s did, from their parents' home to their own instant little nuclear family. And then, of course, it's becoming increasingly clear that with the extension of the active lifespan – the possibility of having to live for twenty to twenty-five years after the death of a partner or divorce – you'd better have a social network.

AGB: So in what ways can our communities be strengthened?

SC: Gosh. I think we should design our communities in ways that give incentives for people of all different ages to be together. For example, you could double-up childcare and recreation centres for older people. Governments could make a big effort at bundling not only their housing complexes but social services in ways that encourage people to interact across generations, even if they're not part of the same family. I think that would be very helpful. I would also lobby to extend family-friendly work possibilities and to give the same time off and flexibility to individuals without kids or ageing parents who would like to volunteer. I would make paternity leave mandatory.

AGB: What can ordinary mothers do to strengthen their communities? You've spoken about middle-class women in the nineteenth century having a moral responsibility beyond their households, an idea I love. Imagine if we all had a real sense of responsibility to our community.

SC: For me, one of the best things women can do for children is to involve men. We need to stop seeing caregiving as a women's issue. We need to develop work policies and work hours that allow men and women to get involved in community activities. I'm very much in favour of "use it or lose it" incentives for men to take paternity leave.

AGB: An incredibly important innovation. I've seen too many cases of career-facilitated paternal detachment, where married fathers walk away from their families without any real sense of loss because their attachment to their families was so tenuous.

SC: Men also feel work and family balance stress. Men also have ageing parents to care for. We need to make men our allies. All human beings have caregiving capacities, and it should be built into our societies to let them carry them out.

AGB: How can mothers train their sons to be good partners?

SC: One thing women have to do for the next generation is to make sure their boys do equal amounts of housework!

AGB: You've written about the decline of child labour changing male perception of children from economic assets to economic liabilities, reducing the economic incentive for fathers to seek custody of their children. What are the social results of this shift in perception?

SC: Mixed, I think. On the one hand, of course, the abolition of the exploitative child labour of the past – both in and out of the home – is a very good thing. It means that we no longer have an economic incentive to have kids just to insure our old age or to add another worker to the family, which weeds out some of the bad reasons to have children and forces us to be more conscious of the sacrifices we must make to raise them. But it also means there are fewer organic bonds between the generations other than the bond of love. And it makes it more difficult to give children a sense that they have an important contribution to make to the family.

AGB: You've addressed the lengthening of what you term "economic adolescence" as being responsible for men's reluctance to marry. Could you elaborate on this?

SC: As education becomes much more important and economic independence becomes something that has to be postponed until you have established a track record – education, jobs – I think both men and women are increasingly postponing marriage for that reason.

AGB: Tell me about the historical lengthening of adolescence.

SC: Even as late as the 1950s, you could drop out of high school without a diploma, find a job pretty easily, and within about ten years be able to support a family. Child labour laws meant that there were fewer and fewer options for a kid other than to stay in school, and the rising educational premium, hollowing-out of middle-class jobs, and de-skilling of traditional occupations meant that increasingly, kids had to stay in school. Adolescence is, I think, really less a biological or hormonal state than it is an emotional one; it's basically a state of suspended animation. People can't develop their executive brainpower unless they're given opportunities to do so.

AGB: What can we do to help our children develop these executive skills?

SC: I believe in giving children responsibilities. Absolutely! I'm in favour of part of the school year being some sort of community work project, and giving them some options in how to do it.

AGB: I wish education departments were so progressive. The two things I would like to see introduced into schools? Both the experiences you mention and the teaching of childcare, from the neurobiology of love to the evolution of the senses and emotional development, presented within a biological, historical and philosophical framework. Imagine how this small act would change the world, not only from an ideological perspective – a formal recognition of the importance of intimacy – but also as an act of supreme pragmatism: teaching our children not only how to parent effectively, but how to understand their own needs and behaviours. The potential for emotional literacy, which is the strongest indicator of success in life, would be staggering. Suicide rates would drop, as would rates of addiction, self-harm, and so on.

SC: Look, there's not an integral role within the family or the community that kids are allowed to play! Old-fashioned child labour was a terrible thing, but having no role – no useful duty to perform – is also a tremendous burden.

AGB: Children are now perceived as little more than entities to be conditioned and entertained.

SC: Yes, exactly.

AGB: There is a massive, monstrous global emphasis on entertainment for the young; music, in particular, has come to assume the dimensions of a religion to adolescents, who otherwise have no sense of purpose within the tribe. The hair, the clothes, the face-paint: tribal markers.

SC: Right, right. My husband's really good at this. He runs a kind of ranch/farm. Kids who can't even reach the pedals on a ride-on lawnmower come out, and he'll put blocks on the pedals and let them mow the field. And they're so happy. It's their idea of summer camp to come and work with us all day! [laughs]

AGB: Bethesda loves the idea of being useful – helping me with the computer, setting the table, making a salad. So how do we restore this sense of purpose in our children?

SC: I think that kids should be reading to their elders or the sick – helping to care for them, helping to feed them; I mean, there's a lot of stuff for them to do. You just have to organize it so that it's not slave labour, not exploitative and not dangerous, which shouldn't be too hard. When my kid was very young, before he could actually do much more than pretend to read but knew the stories by heart, I said: "Listen, I like to cook good food and you like to eat good food, but it's very boring to cook, so every night when I'm preparing food – and this is your job, your responsibility – you find a book and you read to me." And he liked it so much that he wanted to do it more. So he'd take his book to the seventy-year-old couple next door and say, "Can I read to you?" And they loved it, you know? They were very unhappily married, so the only time they ever sat together was when he read to them! [laughs]

AGB: A beautiful solution. In one move, you break the chronological apartheid, reintroduce intimacy, give both the child and old person a sense of purpose and something to anticipate, and it's a circuit-breaker for the TV-PC-CD passive entertainment cycle. If even only some of us did this, we'd see our communities grow stronger. The only care that would have to be taken is to train children to avoid potentially dangerous situations with child abusers.

SC: Kids are not going to take responsibility unless it's given to them. When my son was fifteen years old, I got him to volunteer at an Easter Seal Respite, which is where teen volunteers, along with slightly older paid counsellors, are responsible six days at a time, twenty-four hours a day, for successive groups of severely disabled campers of all different age groups. Two volunteers were assigned to each of the campers. My son hardly slept; he learned to drink coffee; I'm sure he had beer; and the next year, he lost his virginity there. But all those things paled into insignificance against the fact that he came home and said, "Mum, you could never handle this job!"

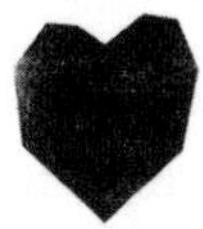

Land of the Spirits

The first death

His incapacitation was temporary, a kind of dream, something like terrestrial existence.

When Bethesda was three years old, my father died. Quietly, in the opening notes of the morning, and before my mother could return to her vigil beside his bed. He had collapsed some months earlier from a stroke that flooded every quadrant of his brain, the very same stroke that would later generate his first meeting with Bethesda. As my father and I had been estranged for close to a decade, he had never met his only grandchild, but when he stopped breathing it was with the knowledge that he was unconditionally loved by one person, however small.

My mother called to tell me that my father had been paralyzed and rendered incontinent, and that he wanted to talk to me before he died. Alexander, Bethesda and I left almost immediately for the nursing home. My father had been flown back on a stretcher from his holiday property, vomiting and attended by a nurse. That day, my baby finally understood what it was to have a maternal grandfather, a man we had never discussed.

There were and are no framed photographs of him in the house.

Bethesda was wearing a red-and-white checked gingham dress, matching kerchief, black Mary Janes and short white socks. Her caramel hair was in pigtails. She had reviewed herself in the mirror before leaving, turning and stumbling a little as she did. Devoid of vanity, she was eager for approval from this mythological figure, this brand new relative. She wanted me to spray perfume on her wrists as I had sprayed it on mine, and she smoothed her skirts in the cab as she asked questions.

"Why can't he move his legs, Mama?" she asked. And then: "Can he stand up? How does he put his socks on? Will he stand up tomorrow? What about on Wednesday?"

The thing that worried her most was that I would also be felled by a stroke. I told her no, that I would live for over a hundred years, that I would be so old when I died that my face would look like a walnut, and that she would be so old when I died and have so many children and such a wonderful husband that it wouldn't matter so much, because her life would be full of love, and then, when it was time for her to die, I would be waiting for her in the Land of the Spirits, a place of tranquil arbours and great libraries.

"Is Nonno Giancarlo going to the Land of the Spirits?" she asked.

I told her yes, and that he would walk again there, so there really wasn't anything to worry about as his incapacitation was temporary, a kind of dream, something like terrestrial existence. (Alex shot me a look during this explanation; I shrugged in reply.)

My heart beat hard as we entered the home. We lost our way, of course; there were so many floors, so many lives close to being extinguished, and my father's room was tucked away at the end of a corridor, and even then, he wasn't there but in a communal area overlooking the balcony.

I always hold Bethesda's hand, but this time it was not so much for her benefit as it was for mine. My father was almost unrecognizable. The remorseless tyrant of my adolescence had metamorphosed into a heap of pale, atrophied limbs. From his throat, those unfamiliar creaks. He was unexpectedly alert (we had reached him during that daily two-hour window of lucidity). I wept, not because I loved him as my daughter loves her father, but because of everything that could have been: this was the beginning of pre-emptive mourning, and informed by the unsaid.

Bethesda, on the other hand, rejoiced: another grandfather!

She shyly showed him her dress after he complimented her, and took, with her whole hand, the single finger he offered. (He still had some movement in one arm.) They had a conversation. She leaned in over the bed rails, assiduously nodding at his every word. Instinctively, she nurtured him, this sick old man, a man who had never really known happiness, reduced to his very scaffolding, repentant in part but mostly unrelenting. In that moment, I saw in her a tenderness and gravitas that left me breathless. She looked like a nurse tending to a dying soldier in a daguerreotype of the American Civil War. The fact that she had never been proximal to sickness was irrelevant; she was unclouded by the understanding of what it is to be unloved, and radiated only patience. His last words to her were on the phone. "I love you so much, Bethesda", he said.

After he died, she was confused. "Is Nonno still in the hospital?" she asked.

"No", I replied, "he's in the Land of the Spirits".

She paused.

"But how did he get there? Did he walk?"

Her eyes were beautiful in that moment.

"The angels flew down and took him", I said.

She frowned. "But how did they get in? Through the windows?"

"They landed on the roof", I said, beginning to smile in spite of myself, "caught the elevator to his room, and flew back up with him into the clouds".

This explanation satisfied her, and she touched my face as I began to cry.

"It's alright, Mama", she said. "Nonno can walk again now."

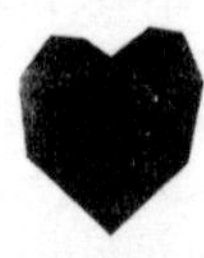

In the trenches

A conversation with Melinda Tankard Reist

The stuff girls put up with!
They don't even know that it's illegal!

Feminist author, advocate, mother of four and self-described "opinionista" Melinda Tankard Reist – known to her friends by the knuckleduster acronym of MTR – is a dangerous woman, as public servant Darryl Adams discovered. When, under a pseudonym on Twitter, Adams jovially asked if anyone had found "naked pictures" of Tankard Reist and described her as "rootable in that religious feminist way", he was complimenting her perhaps in the only way he knew how: as worthy of penetration by a man, if solely on the basis of her righteousness. (Adams was only one of countless detractors, both low and high profile, who denigrate Tankard Reist on the basis of her religious beliefs, if only because it is significantly easier than addressing the points she raises.) Over the following eight months, she hunted Adams down all the way to the Assistant Treasurer. Those who accused her of overreacting missed the point; Tankard Reist was illustrating exactly how normative offensive sexual discrimination has become, and how easily it is cloaked with protestations of parodic intent. Born in 1963, Tankard Reist, the wild, motorbike-riding daughter of farmers, trained as a journalist. She has been offered – and refused – two safe seats from both sides of the political spectrum; her interest is in creating a constituency for change. In 2009, she founded Collective Shout, a grassroots campaigning movement that exposes advertisers, marketers and corporations who objectify women and sexualize girls in order to sell products and services. Tankard Reist's books –

Big Porn Inc: Exposing the Harms of the Global Pornography Industry; *Getting Real: Challenging the Sexualisation of Girls*; *Defiant Birth: Women Who Resist Medical Eugenics*; and *Giving Sorrow Words: Women's Stories of Grief After Abortion* – make her courage and integrity clear: she has never been one to step back from a fight. In particular, she is dedicated to bringing accountability to the corporate sector, which has, over the past half century, identified and exploited – without the slightest consideration of social cost – an inexhaustibly lucrative new market: our children.

AGB: Melinda, tell me about the sexualization of children in this culture.

MTR: We know from a growing body of global literature that children are being increasingly sexualized. They're having adult concepts of sex and sexuality imposed on them at younger and younger ages. Girls are getting a message that they have to be thin, hot and sexy, that their whole goal in life is to attract the male gaze, attract male attention, to be on display. They receive a message that to be female is to bare your flesh – that's how you demonstrate that you are a woman – and so they're not valued for anything else: their gifts, their talents or their desire to make a difference in the world. They're only valued for their sexual allure. Boys are getting a message that that's what women and girls exist for: male gratification and pleasure. They exist to be looked at.

AGB: The ornamental female.

MTR: Yes. Absolutely! To be ornamental is all that women are good for. Tragically, they're getting the message at younger and younger ages, and the research tells us that this is having a raft of negative physical and mental health outcomes. Body image dissatisfaction, eating disorders, depression, anxiety, self-harm, poor academic performance and low self-esteem. When I first started out on this issue, there were only a couple of reports; now there are over a hundred linking sexualization of children, the commodification of childhood and the commercialization of childhood, with all these negative health outcomes.

AGB: Who is to blame? Corporates, pornographers or …?

MTR: Oh, all of the above! Corporates who are looking to expand their markets trying to get brand loyalty from the very earliest of ages. I think you'd be fascinated by the research. A study bankrolled by a group of companies concerned how logos could be embedded into the heads of babies to get babies desiring their brands. And what they did was study drool. They studied the ways babies drool, and noticed that when babies drool, they look down at their drool; they like to watch it hitting whatever it hits, such as their bibs or their jumpsuits. And so the companies worked out that if they could get, say, the Cookie Monster or their logo right where the drool hit, it would become embedded. So they designed the placement of their logos to fit. That's corporate culture.

AGB: Advertising executives are the new Satanists. When Bethesda was one or two years old, I'd take her to the supermarket, sit her in the trolley, and ask her to point out the packaging she found the most attractive. "Pick the prettiest container in the aisle", I'd say. And then I'd pick the container up – usually one with a cartoon emblazoned on the front, or a brightly coloured one – and explain to her why they had packaged it in this fashion. The soft-drinks aisle was always a favourite. "Almost every one of these bottles is full of additives that have no nutritional value", I'd say, "which is why they have to make the bottles so pretty, otherwise no-one would want to buy them. So whenever you see a pretty packet, you can be almost entirely sure that it's full of rubbish. Which is why they put fun cartoons on packaging, because they want children to beg their mothers to buy them. It's very bad." So she got the message pretty quickly. Marketing is a cultural blight.

MTR: Yes it is, and children don't have the cognitive and developmental skills to decipher and screen out the good from the bad. That's why it's having such a destructive impact. I speak to thousands of girls, and it's definitely getting worse. And certainly the pressure that they're under to perform in pornographic ways, to provide sexual favours and sexual imagery … I mean, I've just come back from a school where twelve- and thirteen-year-old girls were just routinely showing me messages that they get: "Send me pictures … I want to see you naked … show me your tits …"

AGB: Are these from boys or men?

MTR: Boys! Just randomly – without being requested – they'll send girls a picture of their penis, with a note: "Now I've sent you a picture of mine, send me a picture of yours. You owe me." These are twelve- and thirteen-year-olds showing me their text messages, having to negotiate and navigate this kind of stuff at an age where they shouldn't have to. Most of them are having some kind of coercive experience. And when you ask them about it, it's so routine. "Yeah, but doesn't this happen to everyone?" They don't see it as unusual to be approached in these ways by boys.

AGB: Of course they don't. Why would they when the general culture supports the pornification of women at every turn? I opened a family newspaper today to find an Italian cartoonist's depiction of Anna Wintour in a variety of sexual positions with Homer Simpson. This was intended as humour. The cartoonist depicted this graceful, high-achieving mother-of-two – now in her sixties – wearing thigh-high latex boots and with her legs in the air. Did Wintour in any way court this level of attention? No. So why is she being presented in this way? Sexualised stupidity. Regression.

MTR: Boy, is it ever! I think this is the most disempowered generation of girls I've ever known. When I ask them about their sexual experiences, they say: "I think I performed okay. He seemed to enjoy it." Totally disconnected from their own sense of pleasure, of intimacy. They don't even think they have a right to be pleasured or to have an intimate experience. They see themselves as sexual service providers. Girls are talking about how boys don't even ask permission to do something – they might be having vaginal sex and then, as the girls report, "He'll try to slip it in the other hole without even asking". Or he'll want to ejaculate on her face.

AGB: I'll never forget a young woman I worked with at a major magazine – tall, heartstoppingly beautiful, very proper – telling me about an eligible bachelor she'd met at a function. He was handsome, charming, erudite and drove a Porsche: the kind of man mothers want their daughters to marry. For the first time in her life, she decided to accept an offer to go back to a man's house. And, after kissing, he paused to politely ask: "Do you mind if I come on your face?" I was incredulous.

MTR: That's right. They'll say, "You're right with anal, yeah?"

AGB: It cuts right across the demographics. I remember overhearing a conversation between two private schoolgirls. "What is with boys these days?" one asked. "They're just not interested in boobs any more – they go straight for your pants." These girls would have been fifteen, sixteen.

MTR: [dryly] Boobs are boring. Even vaginas are a bit boring. Vanilla sex: pffft.

AGB: Let me read you a quote from *8mm*, from Andrew Kevin Walker's film about pornography: "You've got *Penthouse*, *Playboy*, *Hustler*, etc. Nobody even considers them pornography anymore. Then there's mainstream hardcore. Triple X. The difference is penetration. That's hardcore. That whole industry's up in the valley. Writers, directors, porn stars. They're celebrities, or they think they are. They pump out 150 videos a week. A week. They've even got a porno Academy Awards. America loves pornography. Anybody tells you they never use porn, they're lying. Somebody's buying those videos. Somebody's out there spending 900 million dollars a year on phone sex. Know what else? It's only gonna get worse. More and more you'll see perverse hardcore coming into the mainstream, because that's evolution. Desensitization. Oh my God, Elvis Presley's wiggling his hips, how offensive! Nowadays, MTV's showing girls dancing around in thong bikinis with their asses hanging out. Know what I mean? For the porn-addict, big tits aren't big enough after a while. They have to be the biggest tits ever. Some porn chicks are putting in breast implants bigger than your head, literally. Soon, *Playboy*'s gonna be *Penthouse*, *Penthouse*'ll be *Hustler*, Hustler'll be hardcore and hardcore films'll be medical films. People'll be jerking off to women laying around with open wounds. There's nowhere else for it to go." Walker wrote this in 1998. He was clairvoyant. Where do you go when you exhaust every orifice? When every possible combination becomes old hat?

MTR: Well, that's when you get into humiliation and torture and bondage and S&M. Torture porn. Or group. Doctors are telling me as I'm travelling – these are things I'm hearing, things I've never read about anywhere, but this is what's happening: they're treating more and more girls, increasingly younger girls, with anal tearing. Some of these girls are ending up with colostomy bags because of anal sex and even group anal sex. And increasing numbers of oral throat cancer from oral sex in girls. Girls catching the HPV virus from oral sex, thinking oral is safe, and ending up with cancer of the throat. You don't read about those things in the teen magazines.

AGB: I've observed a real push on behalf of the so-called "sex-positive" feminists to rebrand prostitution and pornography as empowering. It's not only socially toxic, but a complete lie.

MTR: Yeah, they've fought hard for their own objectification. It's a false power, and a false sense of empowerment. You might see a handful of exceptions – the pretty porn star with her own website – but let's look at most of the women in the industry who aren't like that. These are the most disempowered of women. Also what was interesting is that many of them had multiple personality disorder. Paedophile ring and prostitution ring owners love those girls, because often one or more of those personas are very young girls, and often clients specifically request those personas. The girls, of course, went into those personas to protect themselves. Comparisons have been made to Stockholm syndrome. These are the only realms in which the girls receive any validation, even if it's the worst kind. "You've got such a great body!", "You're so good at what you do!" and "You're so good at sex – look at the way men respond to you!" Which is why they keep going back.

AGB: A young woman recently uploaded pornographic footage of herself online – for free – to validate her desirability after a friend criticized her body. She said that the response was "totally overwhelming". "I'd like to do it again", she said. "People … said I have to show more flesh to make my posts successful, though. I'll probably do it when I need a pick-me-up." It's heartbreaking that girls now find a sense of confidence not through anything they are or achieve, but by showcasing their genitals. We're reverting to a baboon-like state, if with a sociopathic sheen.

MTR: Yes!

AGB: I was approached through my website by a very young woman who'd worked as a prostitute and then discovered that both her parents had once worked as prostitutes. She's still trying to process what happened to her, trying to understand. She said she was conflicted about the sex-positive feminists using sex workers as their poster girls. "It's empowering on one hand, but on another, it denies their experiences." I included a piece about BDSM sex workers in my first book, *Lunch of Blood*. With the collusion of one of the mistresses, I posed as her assistant – clothed – in session. The sense of entitlement and lack of respect with which the john treated us stunned me; if any office worker were treated in such a fashion, there would be a lawsuit. There was no empowerment in that room, believe you me. The mistress – who had spent her life in and out of psychiatric institutions; who had worked with twelve-year-old girls – was a broken human being. I interviewed a number of prostitutes for that and another story, and they were all dislocated. It's a terrible life, an ancient hangover from the time of slavery. To my mind, the so-called sex-positive feminists are riding into town on the backs of sex workers, and riding them as hard as any john, if in a different way. It's a vicarious exploitation, voyeuristic and destructive. Sex workers are being used as emblems – the phenomenological, emotional or spiritual reality of their existence is of no interest to the sex-positive feminists; all that matters is the concept of choice. Ideas before people.

MTR: I think that's a really good way of putting it.

AGB: Now, I've observed that parents fall into different camps regarding children and pornography. You get our generation, many of whom are unaware of how depraved the material these kids are exposed to can be, right? They literally do not get it. They think it's *Playboy* online, and not autopsy shots, child porn, scatological material, pregnant gang-bangs, violence, rape.

MTR: They think their kids are seeing naked breasts.

AGB: And maybe a vagina or two, and since when did that

kill anybody? Then there are people who believe that it's the parents' responsibility to monitor viewing – as if filters can't be circumvented by internet savvy children; as if children cannot access inappropriate material through friends or the siblings and parents of friends – as I did at the age of seven or so at a girlfriend's house. I don't know what universe these people are living in to think that two working parents can monitor the online and iPhone activities of their children at and after school. It doesn't even make sense. And the third group consists of parents who don't think pornography is a problem – my parents fell into this camp. These are people who understand pornography as synonymous with sex and thus perceive it as healthy or normal or funny. They do not understand how pornography – in particular, how cyberporn – affects the human brain, and how, in particular, it changes the brains of children. I have a lot of information about this on my website. My husband, who attended one of the country's top private schools, had a classmate with a collection of surgical gloves and lubricants for the express purpose of masturbating to pornography. Another pornography fan at his school molested his five-year-old female cousin – this was, of course, all hushed up; the girl's parents were never told. My question is: what are people who care about their children supposed to do?

MTR: Most of the parents I come across feel overwhelmed. It's just too hard for them on their own. As you said, you can have every device monitored at home, but kids are more likely to see it on a friend's phone at school or at a friend's house. And this is why we need proper regulation. Other countries are doing this. The UK has just announced an opt-in system for porn – not to stop adults looking at it, but making them opt in if they want to. Why not? Why do the pornographers want to allow unrestricted access to hardcore torture porn, rape porn, humiliation porn and sadism porn to children? Why is that seen as some great free speech right? This is not an exercise in free speech – in fact, it endangers the fragile right to free speech when you allow it to operate in this way. If men want the right to watch women having their heads kicked in, they can opt in, okay? If they want to see women bound and gagged and tortured and bleeding, let them opt in to that. And yet these men are kicking up a big stink – "Oh, what about our rights!" "Oh, why should we do that?" – like opting in is so hard, you know? No-one's taking it away from you, precious.

AGB: I don't see this as an exclusively male problem. As Belle de Jour – former sex worker Brooke Magnanti's pseudonym – recently said: "The fact that women are porn consumers too is not something you hear a lot about – you're far more likely to hear shock stats about the number of twelve-year-olds looking at porn than adult women, even though the latter category hugely outnumbers the former." This was said in protest against the opt-in system you mention.

MTR: What are these women watching?

AGB: The same things men watch. As romcom darling Kate Hudson, a mother of two, said when asked by a journalist if the porn she enjoyed was soft: "I go right for the hard stuff!" I mean, where do you go when your mother makes statements like this in public? What hope do you have?

MTR: Look, parents need help. It takes a village to raise a child and the village is toxic. We're seeing a rise in child-on-child sexual assaults at a rate never before seen. We're seeing five-year-olds in treatment programs because of their exposure to porn and the behavioural impact it has had. In at least one major First World country, there has been a quadrupling of sex crimes in school-aged young people. A quadrupling in four years! Why isn't that front page news? And all the authorities interviewed said that they attributed this to exposure to pornography. These are the outcomes.

AGB: I spoke at length with a high school teacher's aide. Her report was shocking. Twelve, thirteen-year-olds talking about blowjobs with the laissez-faire of streetwalkers. "It's just sex", they told her. "Who cares about a blowjob? A blowjob never hurt anyone." A friend's daughter who attended one of the country's most elite private girls' schools was set upon at the age of fourteen or so by a gang of the most popular girls who bullied her on these grounds – and I quote – "Your cunt's a weird shape". This is the new bar for girls. All you need is one parent who doesn't care, and their child can infect thousands.

Pornography: a technology-borne pathogen.

MTR: Yes!

AGB: Our gender roles are both reflected and defined by pop culture. Take the hit song *Blurred Lines*: "But you're a good girl/ The way you grab me … So hit me up when you passing through/ I'll give you something big enough to tear your ass in two." And they say romance is dead.

MTR: Girls now see themselves as sexual service stations for men and boys, and boys now believe they have an entitlement to the bodies of women and girls. If a girl resists, she's told that she's prudish, hung up, frigid, that this is what other girls do, and some girls also will say that they'll do what they can to keep this guy, they really like this guy, and so this is what they feel they have to do. They have to pay, with sexual tokens, for a little bit of love. They have to pay for it. You know the expression "friends with benefits"? I remember one young woman asking me, "Why does he get all the benefits and I get none of the friendship?"

AGB: That is so sad.

MTR: Isn't it? I'm not hearing any great, empowered stories about sex from girls at all.

AGB: But what can girls do when they're being assured by sex-positive feminist role models that porn and prostitution are means of empowerment? When academics such as Catharine Hakim encourage them to market their bodies like inanimate objects? Hakim wrote: "If men could produce babies, [surrogacy] would probably be one of the highest-paid occupations in the world, but men ensure that women are not allowed to exploit this unique ability." Exploit this unique ability?

MTR: It's just amazing.

AGB: What I find tragic is that boys aren't being taught to understand sex in context. Sexual conquest – the more mindless, the better – is presented to boys as a subset of masculine prowess; they're made to understand sex in terms of power, of potency, of status. A universe of genitals. Women, on the other hand, have traditionally had sex presented contextually – the end point of a relationship, rather than as a gender identity marker. Sex as inclusive. You've written about the way pornography changes children's views of their own bodies. Can you tell me more about that?

MTR: We know that pornography gives children distorted views of their bodies, relationships and sexuality. They actually come to hate their bodies because they're presented with unrealistic hyper-sexualized ideals, and think that they should look like that. And so a very healthy eight-year-old will say: "I'm too fat." Little girls in primary school will go around pinching their tummies, or pinching their friends' tummies and comparing how "fat" they are. They're playing a compare and despair game in which they always come up short. So, yeah – we're making them sick, basically, and in so many ways. They hate their bodies. It's been said that self-hatred is a rite of passage for our girls.

AGB: So what can we do to protect our children from pornography and sexualization?

MTR: Okay, what I urge people to do is to act personally and act politically. Don't buy into the culture. Don't fuel the demand for sexual slogans on girl's clothing. *Shop somewhere else.* I recommend towardthestars.com for the parents of girls. We have to vote with our wallets. We have to show corporations that we're not going to support them if they don't show social responsibility. And that's where Collective Shout comes in. Contact your MP. Exercise your influence, because mothers have influence. These companies are not going to change unless there's a constituency for change, so we have to create that constituency. It's our responsibility. We have to opt out of a culture that is toxic to our children, and we have to demand something better.

AGB: And how do we teach our sons to respect themselves and women? How do we teach them to integrate their sexuality? Is it a matter of contextualizing sexuality?

MTR: Certainly in the home, there needs to be a zero tolerance policy towards porn. No disparaging sexual comments, nothing. Boys also need to see healthy versions of masculinity, and that's one of the real things I fear. I mean, where do they see healthy masculinity in this culture? Sports stars, heaven help us? We're raising them with a very callous and brutalized version of masculinity, so they don't know how to be good men; they don't see it. Which is why fathers have an even bigger role to play in modelling healthy masculinity.

AGB: But so many fathers are strangers to their sons. Which takes us back to the problem of corporate culture, where fathers – and now, mothers – disappear for up to twelve hours a day. Intimacy is attention-dependent and attention requires time, and who has time these days? Life is crazy. I know of a number of men, some of them high profile, who work absurd hours, return home stressed – and mostly late – watch the news and then look at porn. All married with children. They love the Madonna, but ejaculate over whores. We may as well be living in the Victorian era.

MTR: All these things are interlinked.

AGB: So what are we doing to our children when we tell them pornography is not a problem?

MTR: I think we're engaging in an unprecedented experiment on the healthy sexual development of our children. We're setting them up for failure. And the kids recognize it. They know they're being hurt by porn, but it's compulsive. I'm the one being contacted by thirteen- and fourteen-year-old boys who tell me that they're hooked on porn and they don't know who to talk to. What do I do with all these boys? I can't personally counsel them – that's not my role – but there's nowhere I can refer them.

AGB: And what about schools? What measures should be implemented?

MTR: Three weeks ago, a school principal told me that his school is completely redesigning the toilets. Why? Because of the inappropriate sexual behaviour that's going on in there. So schools are having to do things like redesign their toilet blocks. That's what it's come to! What can schools do? Again, zero tolerance policy. Bring porn to school? Suspension. Download porn on your iPhone? At least a warning, followed by suspension. Not tolerating sexist talk or sexual harassment. The stuff girls put up with! They don't even know that it's illegal! Groping, sexist comments, sexist jokes …

AGB: I remember accidentally interrupting a football meeting in high school – I'd been looking for a debate team meeting. The football meeting had been organized by a young male science teacher, who also coached. I apologized for interrupting, and the science teacher said – I've never forgotten this – "No, stay; we could do with a good hooker." When I told my father, he said he would complain to the headmaster. I told him that I'd handle it myself. When I went to the science master and demanded an apology from the teacher in question, he told me that he'd arrange a meeting. I said, "No, I want him to apologize in front of the whole science staff, otherwise I will take this further". Knowing that the teacher in question would otherwise be sacked, the science master made it happen. So the science teacher was made to apologise before the packed staffroom. He was sarcastic. I said, "I'm sorry; I can't hear you". He was made to apologize again. A beautiful moment.

MTR: How old were you?!

AGB: Fifteen. And I was very angry. So how do we teach our daughters to resist sexualization?

MTR: Again, by modelling it. Don't make negative remarks about your body. Don't ask, "Does my bum look big in this?" Don't work out compulsively. Don't always deprive yourself of dessert. The research tells us that girls take their cues from their mothers, and so mothers have to be really careful about what they say. Try not to always praise your daughter for her looks. Why not praise her for how well she did in her maths test, or how she helped her little brother get ready for school, or isn't it great that she wants to sponsor a child. We need to praise girls for their values, their compassion, their achievements, rather than base our praise on the airheaded cult of appearance. Don't tolerate negative body-talk in the home. Don't buy crap. Get involved in broader grassroots oppositional, transformational cultural movements – like Collective Shout – that will give you strength. I have so many women writing to me saying that it has helped them to be brave.

Melinda Tankard Reist's guide to protecting your children

1. Act personally and politically.
2. Do not tolerate negative comments about sisters or women in general from sons. Fathers have a significant role to play in modelling healthy masculinity in the home.
3. Aim to commend daughters for attributes other than physical appearance/beauty.
4. Mothers avoid comments critical of your own bodies. Research shows daughters take their cues from their mums. If mum doesn't like herself, it is likely her daughter won't either. Throw away the scales. These are a poor indicator of health. Enjoy food. Have healthy attitudes to food and eating as a family.
5. Get your daughters engaged in activities that make them feel good about themselves, e.g. child sponsorship with Compassion or World Vision, local volunteer work. If you can, enable them to spend time in a developing country. This helps them develop a global view and recognize there is a world beyond themselves.
6. Do all you can to build resilience and strength in your child. Establish a network of like-minded friends who will affirm your goals as a parent.
7. Have every possible filtering device on home computers.
8. Have the computer in a public space in the home. Be at least as equally savvy with social media as your children are. Make sure children only have real friends on Facebook and privacy settings set to the maximum level.
9. Don't buy into the culture: don't support stores that sell sexualized clothing, petrol stations where the porn mags are beside the counter next to the sweets etc. Make a complaint directly to the store.
10. Ask your MP/candidate what they are going to do to address the sexualization of children.

Join Collective Shout. This grassroots movement makes it easy for you to understand the issues and make a complaint ("The standard you walk past is the standard you set").

collectiveshout.org

Separated ... with children

On men who no longer live with their families

For much of the twentieth century, 'father' was understood as a fleeting, distracted, nocturnal presence.

On a pale and terrifying morning in August 2007, bestselling British author William Leith awoke to the realization that something was wrong. He was not in a bed, but on an old mattress on the floor. He was not in a house, but in his office. He was alone. He no longer lived with his little boy and the mother of his little boy. Mentally, he was at the end of his tether. Physically, he was fraying at the edges. Bits of him were falling apart.

As Leith was to discover, separation and divorce are now major mental health issues. For the first time in history, households headed by a married couple are a minority in Britain and America, and the numbers in Australia and Canada are decreasing. One in three marriages ends in the first decade; one in five ends within five years (de facto relationships involving children are up to ten times more unstable than marriages). Men aged between thirty and forty-nine are the most likely to divorce, and in over 60 per cent of cases, it is the woman who initiates proceedings (curiously, the bride's age at the time of marriage is the most reliable indicator of marital longevity: the older she is, the more likely it is to last). Mary Eberstadt, author of *Home-Alone America: The Hidden Toll of Day Care, Behavioural Drugs, and Other Parent Substitutes*, calls divorce "the absent father problem".

The emotional fallout extends not only to members of the immediate family, but to following generations, who are forced to deal with the complications and attendant tensions of a single romantic fracture: remarriages, third marriages, stepsiblings and half-siblings, divorce-triggered poverty and social disorganization (changes of residence, fractured communities, and so on). Not to mention the aftershock of separation-triggered emotional problems – difficulties with intimacy, trust, self-image, commitment and depression. *Four Christmases*, the comedy depicting a couple's stressful visits to each of their divorced parents for Christmas, dominated first place in the 2008 US box office for weeks: a poor critical reception did nothing to stifle public identification.

While the normalization of divorce has erased corrosive social stigma – in 1936, King Edward VIII was forced to abdicate in order to marry a "scandalous" divorcee – it has also created a falsely benign image of a process that scars millions of lives each year. In terms of stress, it's up there with the death of a family member. Studies show that positive attitudes toward divorce reduce the quality – and, sometimes, the quantity – of marriage. Social scientist Rebecca O'Neill elaborates in *Experiments in Living: The Fatherless Family*: "This means that, more often, the acceptance of divorce as an option precedes erosion of marital quality, rather than following it as a response."

Researchers and family therapists have known for years that the overall wellbeing of the divorced is significantly worse than that of the married: the evidence is incontrovertible. Despite this, the impact of divorce on fathers is rarely examined, undoubtedly because men are conditioned to contain or ignore anguish and thus regard assistance as emasculating. Statistics, on the other hand, are emotionally eloquent.

After a man divorces, the standard of his physical health plummets, and he becomes vulnerable to anxiety, addiction, depression and mortality (divorced men are 70 to 100 per cent more likely to die between the ages of twenty and sixty than their married counterparts). O'Neill discovered that divorced men are twice as likely to increase their alcohol intake and report the highest rates of unsafe sex (15.7 per cent reporting both multiple partners and lack of condom use in the previous year, compared with 3 per cent of married men, 10.4 per cent of cohabiting men and 9.6 per cent of single men). Nonresident fathers – the most psychologically friable of all divorced men

– are much more likely to engage in high-risk behaviour (drug abuse, drink-driving). *The Journal of Epidemiology and Community Health* reported that separation and divorce more than double the risk of suicide in men.

Those in any doubt about the despair that separation and divorce can engender in fathers need only to address recent headlines. Australian Arthur Freeman, thirty-five, dropped his four-year-old daughter from the West Gate Bridge in Melbourne as her two brothers watched from the car; she later died in hospital, her mother by her beside. Freeman cracked after a protracted custody battle; the night before, he had written himself a memo: "You have a big fight on your hands and by no stretch of the imagination will it be easy."

Freeman's madness is not unique. Englishman Gary Grinhaff, forty-four, bludgeoned his wife to death after she publicly announced their split and then he committed suicide, leaving a note for their two daughters. Aasiya Zubair Hassan, thirty-seven, was found beheaded after she filed for divorce from the 44-year-old father of her two children, Muzzammil Hassan, an American; he has been charged with second-degree murder. Australian Gary Bell, forty-four, gassed himself and his three children: he left a note stating that he could not live without them. Englishman Andrew McIntyre, thirty-nine, smothered his two-year-old son to death before taking an overdose of pills. His suicide note read: "Leon's with me now and no-one can take him away." Scotsman Robert Thomson, fifty, was said to have "reacted badly to the breakup of his 27-year marriage", and stabbed two of his children to death before slashing his wrists. Englishman Gavin Hall, thirty-three, smothered his three-year-old daughter on discovering that his wife had had an affair, and fellow Englishman Christopher Hawkins, forty-seven, stabbed his son to death and attacked his daughter after discovering that his estranged wife had a new partner. Neil Crampton, thirty-six, also from England, butchered his two young children, their uncle and their mother after she said that she no longer wanted anything to do with him.

"I couldn't hack the fact, no", Crampton told the court after five suicide attempts, "she was a beautiful woman; I was losing her like you've said".

In October 2008, Oscar-winning *Dreamgirls* actress Jennifer Hudson lost her mother, brother and her seven-year-old nephew when her sister's estranged American husband, William Balfour, twenty-seven, opened fire on her family (the boy was his stepson). Balfour's psychosis was triggered by his jealousy over Hudson's sister's new boyfriend.

Psychologist Steve Biddulph is familiar with the isolation experienced – and created – by men, and also with the common reaction of rage to feelings of emotional impotence. At the core of the divorce problem, he believes, is a cultural disdain for intimacy. We are, he says, taught to prioritize professional achievement over unhurried time spent with our partners and children, which means that the skills upon which intimacy pivots are a dying art.

"The devaluing of parenthood – mothering and fathering – has harmed us", Biddulph explains, "in that many couples now form with shallow goals: they build an economic union with a sexual commodity. The marriage becomes a shopping-and-pleasure seeking team. Marrying to create a family, with its buzz of sharing, laughing, struggling and sacrifice in order to enjoy deeper pleasures, has diminished. Of course, many people would realize that this is what they want, if they thought about it more deeply. And having this goal would make it possible, and, in fact, essential not to quit when the going gets hard. Because it always gets hard before it gets better."

Biddulph's views chime perfectly with those of Leith, who, in his latest memoir, *Bits of Me Are Falling Apart: Dark Thoughts from the Middle Years*, also addresses the impact of the economy on love. "Look at the world we've created, and how it works!" Leith exclaims. "It's guys who have created it! Discoveries on the differences between male and female brains show that the male brain is all about making things into systems and little machines, and the female brain is about understanding interrelating, and not in a mechanistic way. Men are in trouble. All of our little machines break down, and then we get in a rage about it. Our machines – corporate finance, whatever – are all falling apart.

"What's happening to relationships is the same as what's happening to communities. Because there's simply not enough to go around, people are being forced not to co-operate just to survive, and even though we seem rich, we're not; everybody's mortgaged up to the hilt. When people live in that environment, they become harsher, and harder, and feel worse about themselves, and that seeps into everything – relationships, too. The key thing? People who spend a lot of time making money become money rather than love, as it were. And money is a poisonous model."

The association between fatherhood and finance has, in the last few decades, become almost synonymous. For much of the twentieth century, "father" was understood as a fleeting, distracted, nocturnal presence, and, in many cases, this presence has been further diluted to a weekly event: "Dad" as a species of generous uncle– distant, but kind. GK Chesterton once described family as "this frail cord, flung from the forgotten hills of yesterday to the invisible mountains of tomorrow", but his perception has been crushed by an almost inescapable postmodernist emphasis on consumerism and narcissism: as almost 60 per cent of marriages end in divorce and mothers are, in 88 per cent of cases in Australia, awarded custody, the paternal role has become increasingly complicated to define.

In *Fatherless America: Confronting Our Most Urgent Social Problem*, David Blankenhorn notes that up until relatively recently, fathers were seen as "primary and irreplaceable caregivers", bearing the ultimate responsibility for their children in both law and custom, and responsible for their children's outcome. Predictably, the Industrial Revolution's "progressive fragmentation of labour, combined with mass production and complicated administration, the separation of home from the place of work, [and] the transition from independent producer to paid employee" has resulted in a progressive and emotionally devastating loss of paternal authority and impact on the family.

The many problems created by this new paternal detachment include emotional disengagement from the children, which in turn has led to peer-modulated childhoods and an epidemic of severe behavioural issues in children. Boys in particular have no consistent model of masculinity, and violently struggle with identity. Numerous studies have shown that relationships between nonresident, divorced fathers and their children erode over time, previously intense parenting involvement notwithstanding. Thirty per cent of non-custodial parents have no contact with their children.

There are many explanations for this toxic erosion of affection: difficulties regarding access (finances, transportation, work, maternal noncompliance), devaluation as a parent, lack of involvement in decision-making, the schizophrenic bifurcation of identity (bachelor dad), defensive hostility from the children, and so on, all of which can cause nonresident fathers to withdraw. And for some, the anguish is intolerable. The tragedy? Fathers who have been disengaged from their children for years continue to experience the grief as intensely as those who have only recently lost contact.

Blankenhorn reports that fathers are vanishing legally as well as physically. Almost one-third of US births now take place outside of marriage, and the father is never legally identified in two out of three cases of unwed parenthood. Around 400,000 Australian children live apart from their fathers. In South Africa, single-parent families are now the norm – a mere 33 per cent of children are growing up with both parents. Eight out of ten single-parent families in Canada are run by mothers. And of the two million single-parent families in Britain, a mere eight per cent are headed by men.

Fathers – and the very concept of fathers – are increasingly seen as unnecessary.

Stephanie Coontz, the renowned historian and author of *Marriage, a History: From Obedience to Intimacy, or How Love Conquered Marriage*, agrees. "I think the big problem we have is that neither our economy nor our governmental institutions really value parenting", she sighs. "Despite the lofty rhetoric, they penalize caregiving of all kinds. And they don't value children, especially in Australia and the United States. So children in all types of families have higher poverty rates than, say, in Western Europe. We also have an antisocial definition of happiness, which encourages people to cocoon.

"There have always been fatherless-by-war children, and high death rates have meant that the children of the past, right up until the early twentieth century, were more likely to lose a parent to death before they'd left home than modern kids are to lose them to divorce. That said, there were in the 1980s and 1990s more children affected by divorce than probably at any other time in history. Doomsayers say that having a dead father is less harmful to kids than having a divorced one, but on average, children with stepfathers do less well than children in any other configuration."

Drew*, forty-two, is a forex trader. He idealized his father, who died suddenly when Drew was nine. His mother remarried. Drew hated his stepfather. He has suffered – and disguised – problems with intimacy and addiction all his life. At the age of thirty, he married a woman whose parents had two things in common: their children and multiple divorces. Drew's marriage was poisoned by his wife's fear of confrontation and his scorn (when she asked him why they never made love, he unforgettably replied, "Let's face it, you're no Elle Macpherson"). On 10 September 2001, he received a call from his wife, who was on vacation with their two daughters. Ordered to leave the family home by the time she returned, he lost two million dollars on the market that week.

"I should never have married a woman who doesn't communicate", he exhales. "Yes, I played my part; yes, there are things I would have done differently. Fact is, divorce has sent me broke and into a debt trap I can't get out of. I had to leave London and move back in with my mother in Birmingham. The girls miss me and I've missed out on the best years of their lives. Twenty years ago I was drinking a lot, enjoying myself, seeing women and had no responsibilities; now I have major responsibilities, study part-time, work full-time and never enjoy myself. I'm on a treadmill going nowhere."

Research suggests that however at fault – through infidelity, porn addiction, substance abuse, emotional or physical violence or emotional inaccessibility – most men remain reluctant to accept real responsibility for the erosion of their marriages. This tendency not only precludes the self-awareness that changes destructive patterns (60 per cent of second marriages end in divorce), but has been shown to worsen over time. In this respect, Drew is typical. His adversarial rhetoric, the lingua franca not only of the playing fields but of modern masculinity, is also the hallmark of fractured marriages.

In *The Argument Culture*, bestselling author and sociolinguist Deborah Tannen writes: "[L]egitimate, necessary denunciation is muted, even lost, in the general cacophony of oppositional shouting. What I question is using opposition to accomplish every goal, even those that do not require fighting but might also (or better) be accomplished by other means, such as exploring, expanding, discussing, investigating and the exchanging of ideas suggested by the word 'dialogue'. I am questioning the assumption that everything is matter of polarized opposites."

The wrath and contempt that underscore the adversarial divorce can also kill.

Sam*, thirty-nine, a political science lecturer, found finances to be the least of his problems when he filed for divorce. "We were both professionals", he shrugs. "My greatest fear was for our son, Paul, who endured a consistently angry, miserable home atmosphere at the age of two, followed by the back-and-forth of separation from his mother and the relative strangeness of my bachelor environment. Like all nonresident fathers, I grew apart from my son to some degree. He had problems with anxiety and phobias very early on, and attempted suicide for the fourth time two weeks ago at the age of eighteen, taking an overdose of sleeping pills and painkillers: his eyes rolled back into his head, he had mini-seizures, and slept for fifty-six hours. Although it's entirely against my beliefs in some ways, I think it would have been better for him had his mother and I stayed married. But that may be a guilt-ridden father's fantasy."

When Constance Ahrons, author of *The Good Divorce*, studied 173 children from 98 divorced families, she discovered that the children of parents who remained disengaged from, or hostile to, each other continued to feel damaged even twenty years later. Despite the fact that most children of divorce express a marked preference for unrestricted or increased access to the nonresident parent, researchers discovered that children who have such access are more emotionally disturbed than their counterparts. Increases in the self-esteem of boys and younger children who had frequent and regular visits to their fathers were countered by behavioural difficulties; girls and older children in the same position had fewer behavioural difficulties but lower self-esteem.

Critically, there is the feeling of being secondary. The

adult children of divorce speak of their needs having been sidelined in favour of their parents' work stress, squabbles or anger. Their divorce rate is 57 per cent; the divorce rate of the children of married parents is 11 per cent.

Peter*, twenty-nine, has only seen his parents together once, and that was to discuss a disappointing report card. They divorced when he was two, battled over custody, and retained only the most superficial courtesy in their dealings with each other over the years. His mother, a barrister, allowed him to stay with his father and his new wife every Monday night and second weekend, and Peter was expected to abide by different rules in each household. In effect, he was expected to pretend to be two different people, creating significant difficulties with emotional integration in adulthood.

He pauses before speaking. "Of course I still love my father", he says, "but I also feel let down by him. First, he divorced after only two years of marriage – which, to me, smacks of poor effort on his behalf; he should've sweated it out for longer. I see him as weak. And then he remarried, which I suppose would've been all right if more effort had been made to include me in his second family. I always felt like an outsider. I think a child of divorce is always going to feel that to a certain extent in the second family, but the real problem was that my stepmother and father never did anything with my mother. The two families – my original one and my father's new one – were completely separate, when the bonds between them were, in essence, an elephant in the living room.

"I certainly grew up not trusting men. And I guess I didn't trust my father, either. I didn't understand men – I always wondered if my male friends were using me, or judging me, or just sticking with me because it was convenient. As for older men, I was so uncomfortable with them that I'd often seize up and stammer during conversation. I never challenged them; I just did everything they told me to, and expressed my anger through passive-aggression – messiness, sloppiness, insults behind their backs. But I was always extremely confident with women, and while you hear about a lot of guys having trouble talking to them, I never did. So I guess I held my mother in higher regard. I would certainly never want to treat a woman the way my father treated my mother."

Now married, Peter has watched his parents unite only in their disdain for his wife, replicating the divisiveness that characterized his childhood. "They justify it with rhetoric about her personality, but the fact is that both my parents are incapable of any unity, meaning that once again, I have to be two different people: one when I visit them, and my real self at home with my wife. There is just no way of getting my parents to accept responsibility for their choices; it's all about blaming my wife. The only consistency in their parenting has been the imposition of divisiveness."

In *Marriage, Divorce, and Children's Adjustment*, Robert E. Emery writes of a study of couples randomly assigned to either mediation or litigated divorce. It was discovered that even only five to six hours of mediation had significant long-term effects. It took litigants twice as long to resolve disputes as those who underwent mediation, and even a decade later, the latter group was much more likely to come to mutual decisions about child-related discipline, morality, vacations and academic performance. Mediation also resulted in nonresident parents maintaining much more contact with their children.

Collaborative divorce was pioneered in 1990, and its popularity is growing: the number of professionals involved has, Coontz notes, increased twenty-fold. Despite these notable advances, family law remains an essentially provocative and adversarial system, where former partners are encouraged to degrade and demean the other in order to achieve their goals, whether custodial or monetary. Coontz reported that in 2007, the Colorado Bar Association deemed the process unethical "because it diluted a lawyer's undivided loyalty to the client. Many attorneys still advise divorcing clients that they'd be foolish to give up any potential advantage in a struggle with so many consequences." Not to mention the substantial legal fees that accompany litigation.

Bruce Willis and Demi Moore are examples of the way divorced parents can behave. Their three daughters' feelings have always been their priority, which is why Willis has always made a point of being supportive not only of his former wife's work, but of her next marriage: despite the fact that Ashton Kutcher is twenty-three years his junior, taller and model-beautiful, Willis – bald, simian, ageing – publicly embraced him as his daughters' stepfather. In a 2007 Vanity Fair photospread, Willis fishes from the front of a boat as Kutcher and Moore cuddle in the rear. Willis generously remarked: "It's hard for people to understand, but we go on holidays together. Demi is the mother of my children and Ashton is the stepfather … I'm thrilled that [he] turned out to be such a great guy."

The late Oscar-winning actor Robin Williams also chose the collaborative divorce route, steadfastly refusing to badmouth his wife of nineteen years in public. And hip-hop mogul Russell Simmons, on finalizing custody (and a substantial child support arrangement) with ex Kimora Lee Simmons, noted: "Kimora is a excellent mother and is doing a great job with [our children. They] are studying a couple of foreign languages, they travel around the world, they practise yoga, ballet, swimming, karate and piano … my kids live a tremendous life … Their mother manages all of [it] and I'm happy to provide."

It's an intelligent trend, and one requiring the ability to place the needs of children before all other considerations.

"Divorce is a necessary process as couples do find that they are a mismatch, or have grown in ways that now make them incompatible", Biddulph says. "But my wife and I believe from thirty years of working with couples that about two-thirds of divorces are preventable. Essentially, almost all couples are very immature when they marry or partner. A long process of maturation begins, which involves a great deal of negotiation and learning. None of us has the same marriage we started out with – and thank goodness!

"The crises through which a marriage grows are scary. If partners don't have a strong inner sense of security, as well as kindness and the willingness to listen, then they may panic, blame and attack: the result is a breakup. Couples who work through and keep talking during these tough times usually break through to a higher level of closeness. We all progress from the pretend puppy closeness of young couples, who are largely in love with a projection, rather than a real person. Being able to be close to another person, faults and all, and also having a clear sense of self and not being co-dependent, is a lifetime project. You see this in some old couples –

feisty, passionate, but in no way clingy or into destructive or controlling games. They are a joy to be around."

Leith was unusual in that he not only accepted full responsibility for being dumped, but agreed – in print – with his former partner's reasons for leaving. He used the separation to better himself. Devastated by her (accurate) accusations of monetary mismanagement and immaturity, he organized his finances, lined up book deals, bought his first house, and published what can best be described as an open love letter to her and his son.

"Emotional accountability is really important", he says. "As a kid, you have an instinct to justify yourself, but if something bad happens in adulthood, it's nearly always your fault and you really should face up to that. Forget about expectations of your partner's behaviour – you can't control them, so don't try. I know that if something makes me feel like losing my temper, it's always better not to speak in anger, but to say: Look, we could have a bad row now, and you're not seeing some of what I'm saying, and I'm not seeing some of what you're saying, but let's not go there. In ten days' time, we'll see that we were both fools. It's better to take the longer view because otherwise things can escalate."

Leith's perspective is wise. Research demonstrates that the most common triggers for divorce are lack of communication and affection. The most disturbing findings are that most miserably married adults who divorce are no likelier to enjoy emotional improvements than those who stay married. One study demonstrated that even after a decade, a third of divorced men claimed they would never recover from the pain; almost half admitted to still feeling anger toward their former partners; a high percentage confessed to residual love; and thirty per cent regularly had tender thoughts about their ex-wives.

"A great many people are very immature", Biddulph remarks, "and by divorcing, they often avoid the growth and development of hanging in there and keeping on talking. For your kids' sake especially, you need to work through your differences: keep talking. Men find this hard, right at this point in time because they often have very little language for relating, and this stems from their distance from other men. Men who have been in therapy or men's groups or who have read my book *Manhood* understand the need to be strong but also safe to be around and don't run away or shut down. They find a voice their women can listen to with joy and relief. Because women want strong, gentle men."

* Not their real names.

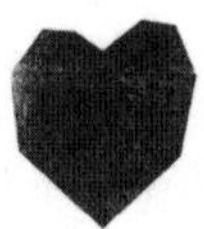

A sacred duty

A conversation with Gabor Maté

The public domain is informed by a culture that doesn't understand attachment, so we're living in a culture that erodes, undermines and interferes with attachment. And increasingly so.

Gabor Maté's face is a narrative of suffering. Sculpted by terror, it is a lapidary series of planes and angles broken only by the black pools of his eyes – eternal in its stillness, more geological than mortal, it compels through its restraint. Often, the only indication of emotion is a change in the pattern of his blinking. His laughter, too, is stifled – so rapid and odd a noise that it could, in different circumstances, be mistaken for pain. Maté was taught to choke emotion in his infancy, when the Wehrmacht and the SS descended upon Budapest, the city of his birth, to deport Jews to Auschwitz. The ensuing chaos determined the course of his life. Now seventy-one and married for over forty-five years to the mother of his three children, artist Rae Maté ("my soulmate"), he is based in Canada and best known as a physician who specializes in addiction, ADHD and child-rearing. Maté has made a point of focusing on the centrality of the early childhood experience to the brain, and how it relates to everything from disease to mental illness. "What I am seeing is the destruction of childhood", he concludes. His bestselling books – *In the Realm of Hungry Ghosts: Close Encounters with Addiction*; *When the Body Says No: The Cost of Hidden Stress*; *Scattered Minds: A New Look at the Origins and Healing of Attention Deficit Disorder*; and *Hold On to Your Kids: Why Parents Need to Matter More Than Peers* (co-authored by developmental psychologist Gordon Neufeld) – are superb; Maté's sweeping intellect and compassion are as engrossing on paper as they are in person. He speaks movingly of "finding the map within ourselves", of evolving beyond trauma into nurturance, and of living rather than just surviving. In essence, Maté expands on the theories of revolutionary psychologist Alice Miller and in that, has changed both the cultural spin on child-rearing and our understanding of addiction. "Genes", he explains, "have a predisposing role, but predisposition is not the same as predetermination". Ultimately, his goal is sacred. Maté's dream is that "people should have full access to the powers that have been given to them".

AGB: Like Alice Miller, you believe that the core of addiction is childhood abuse.

GM: Not just childhood abuse, but childhood emotional loss. Abuse is a specific term. The more hardcore the addiction, the more likely there was a trauma there, but there are people who are addicted who were not abused in the strict sense of the word. As Donald Winnicott, the great British child psychoanalyst, pointed out, there are two things that can go wrong in childhood: one is where things happen that shouldn't happen, and that's huge; but the other is where things that should happen, don't. The loss of what should, but doesn't, happen, can also be very hurtful to the child. So that's the heart of addiction – and, by the way, not just the heart of addiction, but the heart of cancer, rheumatoid arthritis, multiple sclerosis …

AGB: Illness as manifestation of emotional disorder?

GM: At the heart of addiction, mental illness, physical illness and chronic illness is emotional loss, and the more that emotional loss is traumatic in the sense of abuse, the more likely it is going to evolve into cancer, arthritis, mental illness or addiction. So we're talking about a continuum.

AGB: You have said, "If you lose connection with mother, you lose connection with the world". So what happens if this continuum – a continuum of love, of attention – is broken?

GM: In what way?

AGB: I'll use the example of the British serial killer Ian Brady. Moors murderer. Unrepentant. Got off on the sexualized torture of children. Unimaginable stuff. I couldn't even read the reports; they were just too horrible. But what interests me is the genesis of his brutality, the point of fracture.

GM: He was abused.

AGB: It was more interesting than that. His very young, impoverished, single mother – his father has never been identified – used to leave him home alone while she worked. Brady spent days on end by himself as an infant. When he was four or so months old, she had him adopted by a local family. She wanted to spare him the stigma of illegitimacy. So at the most vulnerable time of the human brain's evolution, Brady literally had … nothing.

GM: First of all, I would argue that to leave an infant in solitary confinement is abuse.

AGB: Technically, yes, although I don't think that his mother's intention was abusive.

GM: I understand. She wasn't trying to hurt her child, but it was traumatic for the child nonetheless. In this case, it wasn't that the killer was hit or tortured by his mother, but that what should have happened didn't happen. And what should have happened is the connection. And not just connection, but attuned connection. Brady should have been held, received, comforted, cherished, all that kind of stuff. And when that doesn't happen, the child loses.

AGB: I knew a little girl with Brady's same hypnotically blank stare – those huge, spooky, unblinking eyes. She used to play alongside Bethesda in the park. Her responses were so eerily devoid of emotion that she could seem inhuman. No enthusiasm, no upset. And then her mother, a beautiful, moneyed woman in her late twenties, told me that she had never touched her daughter unless strictly necessary. The only time she ever made physical contact with the baby, she said, was when she was scheduled to change or feed her. So this little baby was left alone, staring at the ceiling, for hours, while her depressed mother sat in the other room, staring at the wall.

GM: Are you familiar with *The Continuum Concept*?

AGB: Jean Liedloff, yes.

GM: Well, what you're talking about in both cases is a break in the connection.

AGB: So why isn't motherhood discussed as a continuum?

GM: I discuss it that way!

AGB: In the public domain, I mean. Motherhood is never presented as a continuum in the public domain; instead, it is presented to us as a series of tasks and burdens.

GM: The public domain is informed by a culture that doesn't understand attachment, so we're living in a culture that erodes, undermines and interferes with attachment. And increasingly so. Human beings were never meant to be parented in nuclear families – it takes a village, right? – but capitalism destroys the tribe, destroys the village, destroys the extended family. You might live in London and your parents might live in Manhattan for economic reasons, right? So we live in a society that breaks attachments, that doesn't honour attachments, a society that then sees the effects of broken attachments and tries to fix the symptoms without understanding the cause. So we see children in school, for example, with ADHD, and we either punish them or medicate them.

AGB: You've been diagnosed with ADHD, but take no medication, is that right?

GM: It is. *Scattered Minds* was the first book I wrote after my own diagnosis. ADHD is not a disease at all, but begins as a coping mechanism on behalf of the child. When there's too much stress in the environment as the brain is developing – and this takes us back to addiction, by the way; the brain is shaped by the environment, in the first three years, especially – then tuning out becomes the self-protective mechanism. This tuning-out then becomes programmed into the brain, and then we diagnose the child and medicate them and try to control their behaviour, instead of asking: What conditions does this child need to develop properly?

AGB: The other day, Bethesda and I caught the school bus together. Thirty or so primary school-aged children boarded. After a minute, their behaviour degenerated to a terrifying degree – they were literally screaming at the back, pouring water on each other, shouting, shrieking, jabbering. The driver had to stop to calm them. I mean, the degree of agitation was terrifying. And it reminded me of your quote: "[I]f you look at … the three millions of kids in the States that are on stimulant medication and the half-a-million who are on antipsychotics, what they're really exhibiting is the effects of extreme stress, increasing stress in our society, on the parenting environment." Not bad parenting. Extremely stressed parenting, because of social and economic conditions.

GM: The example I give is of Windsor, a city known as the automotive capital of Canada. In 2008 to 2009, the number of child mental health visits went up 50 per cent. Why? Because parents were stressed about the slow-down in the auto-making industry, and the kids were being diagnosed and medicated. Which to me epitomizes what's going on. And so, instead of looking at social conditions, family conditions, support for families and support for parents, we're just trying to control children. Behavioural regulation through medication. Kids feel tension. They absorb stress.

AGB: You have also called the idea that addiction is hereditary or genetic "nonsense".

GM: It is.

AGB: So who benefits from the idea of dysfunction as genetic?

GM: The old idea is this: the father is an alcoholic, the son is a heroin addict, addiction has to be genetic. So simple, right? It lets everybody off the hook, because then as a parent, I don't have to look at my own role in creating my child's misery. And I'd like that, because my three kids, now adults, have problems. So if someone gives me a theory – you didn't do anything wrong, it's just genes – I think: "Hey, great! Now I don't have to worry." What makes this idea powerful is that it has a useful social role. And the social role is this: if it's all genetic, we don't have to look at social policy, institutions, schools, medical systems, jails, governments, social conditions and, importantly, we don't have to look at racism. In Australia, for example, which is analogous to Canada in terms of first population treatment and so on, aboriginal people are so much more likely to have addiction in their lives –

AGB: It's a disaster, Gabor.

GM: And it's the same here! My question: In Canada, there were potentially addictive substances before the coming of the Caucasians. There were alcoholic spirits in some areas, peyote, tobacco, psychedelic mushrooms, all kinds of other plants. These were all known and used by the natives, and you know how they were used?

AGB: To facilitate ritual.

GM: Exactly, which is the opposite of addictive use. The essence of addictive use is oblivion: not feeling. Suppressing consciousness. Whereas the essence of spiritual use is more consciousness, heightened awareness, deeper connection. Now, if addiction were genetic, why weren't these people addicted before the Caucasians arrived? And along with the Caucasians came colonialism, oppression, genocidal policies and sexual abuse – especially the sexual abuse of aboriginal kids by their white teachers, which is how sexual abuse became endemic in the native community. It's an absolute scandal. Tens of thousands of them died in these schools. So now you have this high addiction rate in the aboriginal community. There's nothing genetic about it. It has to do with trauma, with experience, with dislocation from their natural ways. To say it's not genetic, of course, leads to the belief that "these people can't handle modern drugs". Another belief that lets everybody off the hook! Then we don't have to look at history, we don't have to adjust our policies, we don't have to look at the ongoing racism that pervades our society. So the genetic argument is very comforting and very, very useful. Unfortunately, scientifically, it's balderdash.

AGB: It's like the foundation of the twelve-step program, which, incidentally, I think is fantastic for one reason: it may well be based on nonsense, but it works.

GM: I'm going to challenge you on that one: what's nonsense about it?

AGB: The disease model.

GM: Well, yeah.

AGB: The disease model is a myth that works. Having been to their meetings – my ex overdosed on cocaine, and was addicted to alcohol and marijuana for years beforehand – I found a lot of common sense in those rooms. Other than the disease model, which needs to be debunked because it feeds into the whole pharmaceutical machine.

GM: I don't quite agree with you. The disease model is accurate to a certain degree, but it is way too narrow for two reasons. One is that the addicted brain, even before it becomes addicted, is already an abnormal brain, because the early trauma and emotional loss changed the brain circuits so it doesn't function as well. Secondly, behaviour – and especially substances – change the brain further. If I define a diseased heart as a heart that is physiologically incapable of functioning in an optimal way, then you can certainly make that case about the brain. You can show it on brain scans; you can show it on various imaging techniques; you can show it biochemically. The problem is that the disease model is too narrow. First of all, because it's aligned with the genetic perspective, and so the assumption is, "If it's a biological disease, then it has to be genetic" – which is false. What's not recognized is that the biology of addiction arises in interaction with the environment and therefore can be undone by interaction with the environment. So to restrict ourselves to the disease model –

AGB: – is to damn ourselves?

GM: Is to damn ourselves. So it's not that I totally disagree with the disease model; there's a validity to it. But not because it's a helpful myth; it's a helpful reality.

AGB: But a helpful myth is a helpful reality; the placebo effect being a case in point.

GM: But the disease model is not a myth! There's some truth to it, but it's a limited truth. If you called it a limited truth rather than a myth, I would agree with you.

AGB: But aren't you talking about damage rather than disease?

GM: It depends how you want to define disease. I don't use the word "damage" so much because that implies a kind of irreversible harm, you know? But diseased in the sense of "dis-ease", you know? And also in the sense of physiologically not functioning optimally.

AGB: Interesting. I've never considered the disease model in terms of neurological damage. The big emphasis is always on the genes, particularly in twelve-step programs. A Narcotics Anonymous member who had been raped by her stepfather from the age of nine once told me that she wished she could write a book about the genetic origins of disease.

GM: I agree with you that twelve-step programs limit themselves to the disease perspective, when what they need to do is address the trauma.

AGB: But trauma is considered irrelevant. All that matters in this culture is the amount of money you earn. How much do you contribute to the economy? That's the question; that's the only question. I have watched people destroy themselves and their families in pursuit of what they understand to be success, which, in this culture, is defined by an accumulation of stuff.

GM: My next book is about how materialism makes us sick!

AGB: One of your most beautiful and terrible statements: children, you once wrote, are "reacting to the broader collapse of the nurturing conditions needed for their development".

GM: Again, what does the child need? We can talk about the specific physiological development of the brain or the healthy development of the child psychologically into a confident, self-actualizing, emergent, creative, trusting, open-minded creature. Or we can talk about what is needed for healthy brain development. And it turns out that whether we're looking at the chemistry of the brain, the microcircuitry of the brain, the self-regulation circuits, the stress regulation circuits, the attentional circuits of the brain, the relational circuits of the brain, or whether we're looking at the chemistry, physiology and connectivity of all those brain systems, or the emotional needs of the child, the conditions are exactly the same: the presence of emotionally available, emotionally consistent, non-stressed, non-depressed, attuned parenting caregivers. That's what every child needs. And when those conditions are not there, the brain doesn't develop optimally, and the child doesn't develop optimally in an emotional sense. What the child develops instead are a lot of compensatory mechanisms, which we then diagnose as diseases or behavioural problems. In 2006, I wrote an article on Ferberization – letting babies "cry it out". For some reason, this article only recently reappeared on the newspaper's website and within a week, it had been downloaded and shared by 56,000 people. What's interesting is the comments left on the site. A lot of anger, precisely because people feel guilty. Whether they admit it to themselves or not.

AGB: You're touching a nerve.

GM: Yes, but it was shared all those thousands of times!

AGB: You said that too many doctors seem to have forgotten what was once a commonplace understanding: that emotions are deeply implicated both in the development of illness, addictions and disorders and in their healing. I don't know if they've forgotten, or if there's just too much money to be made, because if you look at the ever-expanding definitions of mental illness in the DSM-5 [*Diagnostic and Statistical Manual of Mental Disorders*, fifth edition] –

GM: See, I don't think people are that diabolical. There is some of that, and it's easy to show that the pharmaceutical companies conspire [to sell drugs] – that's obvious; we take it for granted. And that some doctors take big bucks to promote pharmaceutical approaches, you know? There have been scandals about that. Easy enough. But I think it's more organic than that. It's organic in the sense that we live in a culture that separates mind from body. We live in a materialistic culture that basically says that the control, acquisition and production of material goods is the highest goal. In a culture like that, it's inevitable that mind and body are separated, because if we saw people as emotional and spiritual beings, we couldn't exploit them the way we exploit them. So what the doctors are buying into is a mindset that's endemic in this culture. They just reflect this culture as members of it. And with the advent of fantastic surgical techniques, powerful and extraordinarily helpful medications – antibiotics and so on – and imaging techniques and technologies, we've relied more and more on the physical modalities and less and less on human intuition. This separation of mind and body goes all the way back to ancient Greece – 2,500 years ago. Then, more specifically, you have to look at the medical profession and ask: Who goes into medicine? Workaholic, driven, insecure people who need the position, need the power, need the income, that's who – people like me, in other words. When I went to medical school, I thought: "Boy, now people are going to respect me!" Why did I need respect? Because I didn't respect myself. And then there's the fact that most people in the medical school are science graduates, people who've never read a poem in their lives except maybe in high school. The medical selection process favours the technical-minded.

AGB: Robots.

GM: Yep. How does a cult indoctrinate members? First of all, you give them a uniform; second, you subject them to authoritarian leaders; third, you separate them from their families; fourth, you take up all their time with cult activities; fifth, you deprive them of sleep … tally it, and we're talking about medical school. In other words: you need stressed candidates and, in some cases, you actually traumatize them. And in order to survive medical training, students have to suppress their awareness of their own stresses. So by the time they graduate, how capable are they of recognizing or understanding or empathizing with suppressed stress in other people? Which is why they then developed a medical system that pays by the piece, so the more patients you see and the more you churn through in your office or operating theatre, the more you are rewarded. Given all these factors, what are the odds? In essence, what I'm saying is that it's not simply the financial conniving. I make good money as a physician even with a totally different perspective. The fear of loss of money didn't keep me from developing a new perspective that started making sense to me. Their resistance is more internal. It's an emotional resistance to appreciating the reality of people because it would demand a hard look at themselves, and that's hard for people to do when they're given all this status and expertise and hosannahs and adulation. It's very difficult to give that up.

AGB: You were hardwired for stress in infancy. The German army, the Wehrmacht, along with the SS, descended upon Budapest when you were only weeks old. Your mother rang the paediatrician because you wouldn't stop crying. "All my Jewish babies are crying", he told her.

GM: I was born on January 6, 1944; in the January of 1945, the Russians expelled the Germans from Budapest and we were liberated. So that was the first year of my life. I never made it to a concentration camp. They deported the Jews of Hungary in a petal fashion – moving in from the periphery. So they deported half a million people in three months, including my grandparents, who were sent to Auschwitz.

AGB: Did they survive?

GM: No, no – they were gassed. And the guy who sent them there, the Hungarian who collected Jews and sent them in his cattle cars to Auschwitz, died this week at the age of ninety-eight. He was about to face trial for what he did during the war. [pauses] So my mother and I lived in Budapest. My father, a furniture maker, was in forced labour. From the time I was three or four months old to the time he came back a year later, my mother didn't know if my father was dead or alive. What she did know was that her parents had been killed in Auschwitz. The day her parents were sent to Auschwitz, her breast milk dried up. And then came the ghetto. In June 1944, there was such a universal outcry – in the States, in the Vatican – that the Hungarian government stopped the deportation of Jews. So that's why we weren't sent to Auschwitz. But conditions in the ghetto were terrible; you can just imagine.

AGB: You wrote: "No great powers of imagination are required to understand that in her state of mind, and under the inhuman stresses she was facing daily, my mother was rarely up to the tender smiles and undivided attention a developing infant requires to imprint a sense of security and unconditional love in his mind. My mother, in fact, told me that on many days her despair was such that only the need to care for me motivated her to get up from bed. I learned early that I had to work for attention, to burden my mother as little as possible, and that my anxiety and pain were best suppressed."

GM: Yes. And then came several months of right-wing fascist rule, where more people were killed – daily killings and all that – so that was my first year of life. And that included also a two-week separation from my mother; she gave me to a total stranger, hoping I'd be looked after, because she thought she was going to die. Even now at the age of seventy, I'm capable of withdrawing emotionally into myself when my wife and life-partner of forty-five years says something that I momentarily perceive as hurtful, even when, really, it isn't. If my wife and I have a fight, say, my automatic reaction is: "Okay, I'm out of here! You can have the house, as much money as you want, just tell me what the terms are – let's just split, you know?" Detachment is very deeply ingrained in me because of that two-week separation, you know?

AGB: I find your all-encompassing compassion shocking in the circumstances. You remind me of Bruno Bettelheim.

GM: Why does my compassion surprise you?

AGB: To have endured so much suffering and yet be able to alchemize it into beauty.

GM: Okay, so first of all, a few things about that: you've surely heard the saying, "To understand is to forgive?" Once you truly get it, it's like Jesus says, "Forgive them, for they know not what they do". Because so many people really don't know what they're doing. They're unconscious. Some of them may be conscious in their actions, but they're unconscious in the face of their drives.

AGB: Which brings us back to parenting. You've noted that the dominant bias in understanding children is that the problem is behavioural. What can we do to change that prism?

GM: What if we actually got the meaning of the expression "acting out"? You act out when you don't have the language to say something in words. In a game of charades, where you're not allowed to speak, you have to act out. So we need to understand that a child's behaviour is very specifically acting out – then, instead of worrying about the act, we worry about the message. What is being said here? In other words, if you understand the child's behaviour as a manifestation of some internal dynamic and always, always, always a cry for help, it changes everything.

AGB: If you could wave a magic wand, what would you do?

GM: The magic wand would be to see the emotional reality behind the behaviours. And to respond to the emotional reality rather than the behaviour.

AGB: If I could wave a magic wand, I would overhaul corporate culture.

GM: Everyone's overloaded. Stressed. To a significant degree, the problem of corporate culture is out of the hands of any particular individual. We're looking at major cultural, economic and political factors here. There is no magic wand. So that's the first thing. The second thing is this: all any of us can do is keep speaking the truth in the face of what this culture does.

AGB: A major issue is the feminist promotion of child-nurturance as a "choice" for mothers, as if the foundation of a human being's emotional life were on a par with professional status.

GM: Feminism has many important and essential, crucial things to say, but the one mistake they did make as a movement was their take on child-rearing and the importance of attachment. As a result, child-rearing became understood as a mechanical thing that could be done by anybody, anywhere. Feminism certainly got it wrong there, there's no question about it. I remember an interview on *60 Minutes* with an ageing feminist scholar, who said that lawyers and academics who decide to take time off from work to be with their newborns are "betraying everything we worked for. You're allowing yourself to depend on a man", she said, and so on. It was sad to see.

AGB: Men, too, have forgotten that they have to care for women, not simply desire them – in particular, they have to care for the women who bear their children. One of the most tragic facets of our culture is that men have come to understand their role as one of earning money and little more. Loving interdependence has been eroded by the corporate model. The same ideology is evident in pornography, where women sexually service men rather than make love with them. It's the opposite of union, and you can see this played out in so many divorces. I've known men who don't see any conflict in behaving in an openly contemptuous or indifferent way to former partners while simultaneously seeking the approval of the children they share. This cultural contempt for mothers could not be more pronounced. As the aptly named Spencer Pratt said of his mother-in-law: "She didn't make Heidi [Montag, his wife]. She's just a vagina."

GM: Exactly. And then the men demand equal access and all that kind of nonsense. I've seen that many times, too. To be fair to the man, what's happened is that the support of the mother – from family, from community – now exclusively falls to the father. And it's just too much for the husband to deal with. You know, if I could live my life over again, I'd drop my concerns about building a practice; I would have faith that as a physician, I would never allow my family to starve and I would spend time at home with my kids and my wife. If I could live my life over again.

AGB: You seem intensely regretful. Where do you feel you failed?

GM: Let me give you an example. The week that we moved into our present home, when our children were six and nine years old respectively – our daughter hadn't been born yet – I took on fifteen pregnant women for delivery that month. Now, this was in addition to a full-time family practice. So I was always exhausted, half my nights were spent away from home, and what shape was I in when I was home? I'd just moved, had two young kids and a wife who needed my support.

AGB: So why are you still married?

GM: A journalist asked George Harrison's wife the secret for the longevity of their marriage, and she replied, "Not to get a divorce". [laughs] My wife didn't leave for two reasons. The bad reason was that she was too insecure. And there were times when, really, it would have been healthier for her own sake – and for the sake of the children – not to leave me, but to say: "Enough of this! Either you wise up, or we can't sustain this relationship." The good reason is that we tremendously loved each other, were dedicated to working on our marriage, and we had the soul-purpose, the soul – s. o. u. l – purpose of finding the truth of ourselves within the context of our relationship. So that's why we stayed together. I can tell you that without the second purpose, the first would not have worked.

AGB: Even in only a decade, my husband and I have weathered extraordinary storms. Sometimes I wonder how the marriage has survived. He assures me that ours is a great love story.

GM: People marry other people who are exactly at the same level of emotional hurt as they are. So even if the external circumstances look different, the internal emotional charge that they carry is absolutely even; if it wasn't, they wouldn't be together.

AGB: You understand this, and yet you still feel guilty about the mistakes you made with your children. So what do we do with guilt? What should a mother do when she experiences guilt about her mothering in relation, say, to something she has read? How can that guilt be made to work for her?

GM: If you're driving a car and inadvertently you drive over a nail and you get a flat tyre, what do you do? How much guilt do you feel?

AGB: None.

GM: Right. Because you did it inadvertently. You caused some damage – you created a problem – but you didn't do it deliberately. No mother in her right mind wakes up and says, "How can I screw up my kids today?" Mothers damage their children because of cultural pressures, because they don't know any better, because that's how they were raised themselves, because of economic necessity.

AGB: And so what do we do when we inadvertently hurt our children, and they become defiant?

GM: You have to recognize that your child has suffered an attachment wound, and that these behaviours are a reflection of his defences against that wound. The way to help him is to heal that wound. How to heal that wound is to give him precisely what you didn't give him in the first place, which is unconditional loving acceptance, attuned presence and support. I deal with all this in *Hold On to Your Kids*. Your child is not broken. There is neural plasticity, so the brain can change. People, even after terrible abuse, can heal and become whole again, because that wholeness is their birthright. So it's a question of realizing that you did your best, whatever your best was, and just saying, "Okay, what can I do now to repair whatever I inflicted and to rebuilt this relationship?" That's always possible. In other words, it's never over.

AGB: But what about cases of hardcore abuse? Couldn't paedophiles and violent parents use your words as ammunition – that is to say, that their actions have had no real impact? Aren't all the addicts, ADHD sufferers, and so on you see evidence that millions of children are broken?

GM: Anyone can use anything as an excuse. And to say that ultimately you did no damage is not to say that you didn't create suffering or pain, so it's not an excuse for ongoing hurtful behaviour. It's a matter of getting people to realize how the imprinting they received as children has been unconsciously passed on to their own. It's not personal. It's not deliberate. It's a matter of taking responsibility. We all do our best, but our best is limited by our level of awareness.

Gabor Maté's guide to a well-lived life

1. Know yourself. Work on unresolved emotional material.
2. Be intentional. Think out what your goals are for family life and your children's development.
3. Keep checking your lives in the light of your intentions.
4. Put the health and emotional security of the children above all considerations of career, wealth and so on, especially in the first few years.
5. If either parent can stay home with the children in the early years, even at an economic cost, do it.
6. Neither physical nor emotional caregiving should be the job of one parent only, if there are two in the picture. Share caregiving as much as possible.
7. Look after yourself. Your stresses are inevitably transmitted to your kids.
8. Family time should be sacred, such as family meals and weekends.
9. Keep the digital media and screens of all kinds out of the house or as far away from the kids as possible, until they are older and so well-connected to you that they will follow your directions and expectations.
10. If you have a spiritual path or mindfulness practice, keep it up and share with the children in an age-appropriate fashion.

gabormate.com

Why I don't own a television

Life in the slow lane

Television was not to blame for my family's disintegration, but it is, by definition, a facilitator of detachment.

When I remember my childhood, I do not so much remember the climbing of trees (although some trees were climbed), nor do I remember picnics or baseball games because there were none. The parameters of my childhood were determined not by parental involvement, but by its deficit. My father had little time for me and my mother was also unavailable, if for different reasons: where he was hamstrung by obligations, she simply lacked interest. And as a result, my brother and I were mostly parented by television.

It was only after my father's death that I learned his childhood nickname ("Dice") and the matrix of his corrosive fascination with money, and that was only because I had given him a memory book to fill in for his only grandchild. Do you know any stories about the time leading up to your birth? How did your parents choose your name? As I read these questions I experienced a thrill, shot through, as it was, not only with the curiosity of all children of mysterious fathers, but with hope for some kind of abstracted connection, one encompassing a safe distance, resistant to insult, a union that could somehow exist independently of each long-estranged party, both of whom, in the end, may even have been unaware of its existence, or perhaps simply pretended to be.

Unsurprisingly, most of my father's answers were monosyllabic – yes, no – and written by my mother, as his right hand had been disabled by a stroke. Reading the few pages that he had completed made me realize that parent–child estrangement is not only commonplace, but that sometimes it is the only option in the circumstances. My businessman father rose, unseen, at dawn for work, was gone all day and in the evening I shared his incomplete attention with my mother, brother, pastasciutta and a green tureen of table grapes for half an hour over dinner; after that, the television owned him.

Since the 1950s, childhood has been experienced in the interstices between broadcast programs, and in this respect I was an ordinary child; real life was something like the interval during which bladders were relieved and limbs stretched. On our return from school, my brother and I would load trays with snacks – our palates, regulated by copywriters, craved stale concoctions of sugar, salt and saturated fats – to roost on the television-room sofa, an unyielding monstrosity upholstered with vinyl the red of unoxygenated blood, and this is how we spent most of our afternoons: chewing, staring. That screen was a portal. Little more than a curved glass faceplate framed by injection-moulded plastic, it bewitched us as efficiently as a malevolent spirit, with the inexorability of antimatter and no intention, or capacity, to return those lost afternoons.

Reruns of immortal, corny and, in some cases, seminal, sitcoms determined the framework of our aspirations. This parallel universe ran along the rails of our passivity. My brother and I sat as if shot through the head, our critical minds dazzled into dysfunction by the rapid interplay of image and instruction. In time, our dissociation from our other world – that dreary universe of resentful mothers, maths homework and a sun that seemed to burn through bone – was close to complete: even when confronted by our very own resentful mother, we were almost entirely absent, dreaming of wiggling our noses like Samantha Stephens to make her vanish, or of borrowing Major Tony Nelson's bottled sprite to the same end. Our mother never did vanish, but we kept on watching.

Like a family member, our television featured in a disproportionate number of my childhood memories. I first menstruated during a rerun of *Trinity Rides Again*. My brother almost choked to death on a grape while we watched *Wacky Races*. I scorched half my eyebrows off during an episode of *Gilligan's Island* (an unfortunate experiment with a kerosene heater and a candle). One of the few arguments I can recall having with my father – most are no longer accessible, a self-preservation mechanism – was conducted over the televised soundtrack of *If …*, the bleak R-rated precursor to *O, Lucky Man!* (my father, bored, repeatedly ordered me to stop blocking the screen).

On summer nights, my brother and I would crouch on the living-room balcony, our backs to a great valley and that eternity of stars, as we trapped quivering looper moths with our moist, cupped hands. The dust those subtle creatures shed – iridescent, infused with the properties of flight – we understood as valuable, but only within the context of beauty; however thick in application, it would never help us fly. Our parents, separated from us by screen doors, had no interest in any of our adventures. Waxen in that blue-green aura, they were excused from reciprocity of any stripe and silent, reduced – like victims of locked-in syndrome – to the function of vision. Other than a few words exchanged before and over dinner, we had said absolutely nothing to each other all day.

The sharing of trauma can establish intimacy, as survivors of wars and aircraft crashes will attest, but intimacy is generally meandering, the stuff of casual confidences, words seemingly secondary to their subject or context, spoken in idleness, punctuated by unrelated observations, exclamations and ancillary buzz. The intention to be intimate is, in some cases, not even essential; unregarded, intimacy can become an oak, unshakeable: all that is required is an open heart.

Those who deride such exchanges as trivial do not understand their value, for communities are founded on the barter and bestowal of incidental information. The erosion of familial and related intimacies has engendered a need only superficially met by social utilities such as Facebook and Twitter; the illusion of closeness is supplied, without the presence by which love is universally understood.

If television can be said to have a nature, then it is to intercept such conversations and, in the process, dislodge intergenerational attachments – our ties to the past, our ties to the future – by creating a single centralized bond: that created by the experience of watching television. Generations are now united not by communication or direct experience, but by the passive – and emotionally removed – observation of strangers, who are, for the greater part, performing, even in the context of "reality" television.

I do not remember a single day of my childhood as free of television. That vaguely extraterrestrial phosphorescence created a kind of membrane within which we felt protected from the disappointments of the world. But in the place of metamorphosis, dehumanization. Those hours of watching rolled into years. Four hours a day, seven days a week, fifty-two weeks a year amounts to one and a half years of solid television-watching over a decade. One and a half years.

Bit by bit, we broke away from each other and, like ice shelf fragments, gradually – and permanently – drifted in different directions.

Ultimately, my parents owned five televisions and in this respect, were ahead of their time: Nielsen Media Research reported that the average home now has more television sets than people. Any evening, my mother, father and brothers (another brother – unplanned – arrived when I was twelve) could each be found in different rooms, their consciousness of the world receding. Walking through our corridor at night, a corridor I had, with the hallucinogenic brio of all eight-year-olds, petitioned to have painted lime green, was something like penetrating geologically arranged strata of sound: that of Formula One, rape, standup, earthquake, bypass surgery. (My family was not partial to period drama.) Divorced from their visual sources, these vibrations amassed into a low-level dissonance remarkable only for its familiarity: the soundtrack of my isolation.

By this time, I had stopped watching television. The first stirrings of rebellion took place at an indeterminate point between my last manipulation of a skipping rope and first reading of Anaïs Nin, but the repulsion was sudden. I had, as if in a vision, seen myself as I really was, conveniently silent on that red vinyl bier: Disney's Snow White poisoned under glass, or Damien Hirst's gilded calf, nicely submerged in formaldehyde.

Television was not to blame for my family's disintegration, but it is, by definition, a facilitator of detachment. And I was tired of pretending that we were normal, that we were happy, that every situation had a resolution. Rome was burning – the old had been abstracted to memories in the uproar; children, to the sum of their screaming – but at the very last, despite it all, and like Nero, the last Emperor of the Julio-Claudian dynasty and our sober old Alsatian's namesake, my parents continued to fiddle. (Or, as violins would not exist for another thousand years, something like it.)

I no longer wanted to be inert, distrait. The immersion required to enjoy television blurs rather than strengthens the sense of self, and on more than one occasion, I have found myself questioning the integrity of a memory: was it mine, or did it belong to a character on television? The prospect of experiencing life as a three-dimensional event, a narrative, with all my senses, seduced me. Because television, experienced regularly, close to indiscriminately, can only be coarsening. Even the consumption of truffles while watching television becomes secondary to the experience of watching television, reduced to a mundane, an adjunctive, behaviour, which is, perhaps, why the most popular television-watching foods are never savoured when the palate is alert, for fear that their oiliness or staleness or sharp laboratory aftertaste will be made evident and with it, an awareness of the food's failure to function in any nutritional capacity.

More than anything, I was tired of being a member of the audience.

In adulthood, the fact that I did not own a television could, like no other piece of humdrum information, startle. It became clear to me that not owning a television was a radical act, a real gesture of defiance, and that in combination with my work – as a writer, I am expected to intuit the most diaphanous of cultural shifts – it suggested a potentially dangerous disregard for convictions that many hold as closely as their wallets: not concerning democracy or freedom, but the sovereignty of image. Television may have evolved into the organ of our cultural conditioning, that place where, in the absence of consistent parenting, we learn to be human, but that does not mean that it is good. If, in fact, we address the violation of the natural world, and I include human beings in that category, it is clear that our time, at least in part, would be better spent addressing reality.

During my interview with a major television executive, he

noted that when ratings revealed that millions had watched a certain show, he asked himself what the rest of the population had been doing. This man perceived a preference for human interaction as a personal failing. To him, Nielsen's 2009 findings that 18 to 24-year-olds watch an average of 3.6 hours of television per day was shocking – not because the findings reflected the intellectual, spiritual and emotional curdling of the young, but because the demographic watched almost an hour less than 35 to 44-year-olds in the same time frame. What was he doing wrong?

One of my proudest moments as a mother was when I took Bethesda, then two-and-a-half-years-old, to a private maternity ward where a friend was half-watching a soap on the overhead monitor as she breastfed her newborn. Perplexed, my daughter turned to me. "Mama", she said, "what's that box with pictures in the air?"

My girlfriend was dumbfounded by the comment, but I held my daughter close, content.

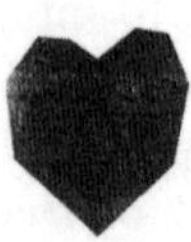

The needs of the mother

A conversation with Michel Odent

Physiologically speaking, women are losing the capacity to give birth, and they are also losing the capacity to breastfeed.

Michel Odent's impact on the world has been immeasurable. The rakish, intellectually electric French obstetrician and founder of London's Primal Health Research Centre was responsible for both flagging the critical importance of oxytocin (the "hormone of love") and introducing the concepts of home-like hospital birthing rooms and birthing pools to the world. Now eighty-four, he has authored close to a hundred articles in medical journals, including the first piece applying the "Gate Control Theory of Pain" to obstetrics (1975) and the first piece about the initiation of lactation during the hour following birth (1977). He is, in short, a visionary, and his work has had a unique role in shaping modern obstetrical practice and midwifery. Odent's twenty-two ground-breaking books – some philosophical, some pragmatic – include *Childbirth and the Evolution of Homo Sapiens*; *Birth and Breastfeeding: Rediscovering the Needs of Women During Pregnancy and Childbirth; Birth Reborn: What Childbirth Should Be; Primal Health: Understanding the Critical Period Between Conception and the First Birthday*; and *Childbirth in the Age of Plastics.* Born in Bresles, a village 80 kilometres north of Paris ("The American soldiers called it 'Breastless'"), Odent enjoyed a childhood dominated by his adoring, intellectually radical mother. Even the Second World War failed to dampen his spirits. Soon after becoming a surgeon, he was put in charge of both the surgical and maternity units at Pithiviers state hospital from 1962 until 1985, and it was here that his fascination with the matrix of human being shook him awake. He remains a provocateur, and very French. "It's not simple", he sighs when asked if he is married. "I am still officially married, but I also had a child in London with an English mother. We co-parent; that child is now twenty-eight. My wife in France and I co-parent, too – our daughter is fifty-five, and she has three children who are adults, so I have three grandchildren. I am based in England, but travel so much that I am everywhere!" And he is, if only in practice. By changing the way we are treated when we give birth, Odent changes our lives.

AGB: Clearly, you were deeply attached to your mother in childhood.

MO: My mother, Madeleine, was in charge of a nursery school in the national French educational system. Something a little bit important: my mother was born in 1895, and was highly influenced by Maria Montessori. Nobody in France had heard of Montessori, but a lady from the USA – Miss Cromwell – came to Paris to talk about Montessori's work just after the First World War, and my mother was one of the first in France to become aware of this approach. She was asked to create a Montessori school, but thought it was better to introduce Montessori's perspective into the national educational system.

AGB: So, like you, your mother was a radical?

MO: She was interested in this new perspective, yes. She was progressive!

AGB: And your father?

MO: My father was an accountant in the local sugar mill. The mill was the main economic activity in the village. Our life together as a family was quite simple – just my father, mother, me and my brother. I started going to the nursery school with my mother when I was two. Our house was attached to the school, so I was following my mummy to school. I remember my mother playing the piano, things like that. The Second World War was the big event of my childhood. We were evacuated to the South of France, we came back … bombardments, things like that. Being born in 1930, I have a very precise memory of this period. To go to secondary school after the German occupation, I had to ride 26 kilometres a day on my bike. There were no cars. A different lifestyle. What I remember from this period is not always negative, you know? We were going to the swimming pool with the German soldiers. Soldiers are all the same, no matter which country they are from. American, British.

AGB: So you don't associate fear or terror with the Second World War?

MO: Not so much. There were difficult times. In 1944, five local people were killed by bombardments. My first experience of aggression was at primary school, even the last year of nursery school, not at home. My young brother often had health problems, you see, so my mother was always busy taking care of him; he was very fragile. I was much more the stronger one.

AGB: So your mother was also nurturing.

MO: Oh, yes! Yes! She believed that early experience has the most profound effect on a human life – that's why she worked in a nursery, rather than primary school. My mother thought that what happened in a nursery school was far more important.

AGB: What did you understand of motherhood when you were little?

MO: Quite simple. Your mummy is a typical protective person, someone you can rely on. My parents had a simple marriage. They spent their life together until they died. My mother died at ninety-eight.

AGB: Tell me about your own understanding of the maternal paradigm.

MO: I was educated as a surgeon. It was via the caesarean section that I became gradually more interested in childbirth, and then I shifted from surgery to obstetrics. I understood the importance of these issues quite late in my life – I was in my thirties.

AGB: What changes do you observe in mothers today?

MO: There are some very practical observations. Physiologically speaking, women are losing the capacity to give birth and they are also losing the capacity to breastfeed. That, to me, is the primary phenomenon. As a race, we are weaker, starting from that.

AGB: You've said that on a planetary level, the number of women who give birth to babies naturally – that is, as a result of an unimpeded oxytocin system – is becoming insignificant.

MO: Yes, which is why I believe that the human oxytocin system – oxytocin being the hormone of love, fundamental to birth and bonding, even in adulthood – is growing weaker. There are two studies demonstrating this: one is an American study concerning the declining capacity for empathy. A huge study, from 1979 to 2009 – a synthesis of seven different studies. That was very significant, you know. The other one I find interesting concerns the duration of the first stage of labour. After taking into account many variables, such as body mass index, and so on, they found that, on average, the duration of the first stage of labour in birth was 2.5 hours longer in 2002 to 2008 than it was in 1959 to 1966. This is enormous. To me, this demonstrates the obvious: that women are losing the capacity to give birth. Yes, doctors have a role through the recommendation of caesarean sections, but women are losing the capacity to give birth. These two studies are a reason to anticipate a weaker oxytocin system in the future.

AGB: Medical ethicist Dr Anna Smajdor recently announced in the journal *Clinical Ethics* that compassion "is not a necessary component of healthcare, since the crucial tasks associated with healthcare can be carried out in the absence of compassion. One can remove an appendix without caring about the person it is taken from, empty a bedpan without caring about the patient who has filled it or provide food without caring about the person who will eat it."

MO: Yet another example.

AGB: When referring to this weakening, you describe human beings as ecosystems?

MO: I use this term to explain the microbiological revolution. It's a new understanding of Homo sapiens – something people have not realized until now. Each of us has in our body more microbes than there are human beings on this planet. We all have in us microbiomes: a community of micro-organisms. So Homo sapiens can be described as an ecosystem. There is constant interaction between your microbiome – the trillions of microbes that colonize your body, in particular the gut and skin flora – and your own genetic materials. There are ten microbes to every one cell, so there is constant interaction, co-operation, symbiosis. Which is why I can talk about an ecosystem. It's a balance, you know, between the activities of the microbes and activities of the cells.

AGB: Tell me about the bacteriological perspective.

MO: The bacteriological perspective is the easiest and most useful perspective to explain to anybody – in particular, medical people – the deep importance of what happens at birth. Today, for example, we understand that our gut flora is 80 per cent of our human system, which means that our behaviour is influenced dramatically by our gut flora, by our microbiome. Gut flora is established immediately after birth. To be born is to enter the world of microbes. So what happens at birth from a bacteriological perspective is much more important than we could have imagined twenty years ago.

AGB: And how does this relate to illness?

MO: We now know that the microbiological perspective explains the increased incidence of some pathological conditions – autoimmune disease, allergies, the dysregulation of the human system. Epidemiologists detect bacteriological risk factors for all these conditions at the time of birth. So thanks to the bacteriological perspective, we finally have interpretation we can understand. The importance of childhood can now be understood from a bacteriological perspective. Up until very recently, the first microbes entering a baby's body were from the mother's perineal zone; it was like that. But today, many babies are not born via this route – they are born via c-section – and that is very serious. And a great number of babies are exposed to antibiotics, and all of that interferes with the gut and skin flora established at birth. This is incredibly easy to explain to doctors; what is more difficult is to talk to natural childbirth groups. They have been repeating the same things for fifty years. Often, they have no scientific background. Natural childbirth groups are not interested in scientific advances, so it's difficult to explain what is important.

AGB: You have spoken very beautifully on the evolution of the capacity to love.

MO: An important topic. A month ago in London, I participated in a conference about human evolution. In fact, I spoke mostly about the future; all the other speakers were talking about the past, all of them – palaeontologists, archaeologists, evolutionists. I said: "Let's talk about the future! The phase of human life that has been most dramatically changed over the past decade is birth – which is, according to the modern scientific perspective, a critical period in the formation of human beings. So let's look at that. We can, in the near future, anticipate a transformation of Homo sapiens." And I jumped on what an evolutionist had said before I spoke – he had repeated what people have said for a long time, which is that since we separated from the other members of the chimpanzee family, the size of the human brain has been gradually increasing – a bigger, bigger, bigger, bigger brain, limited only because the size of the birth canal is an evolutionary bottleneck. This bottleneck ensures that a tendency toward an increased head circumference cannot be transmitted to the next generation. It prevents a steady encephalization quotient. But with the c-section, the bottleneck has disappeared. Now there is no limit to a tendency towards an increased head volume in the next generation. So we can anticipate in the future an increased average head circumference – and an increased encephalization quotient. And then there is the future of the human oxytocin system.

AGB: Michel, that is deeply disturbing.

MO: Yes! Until now, when thinking of evolution, we are only thinking about "hard inheritance" – that is to say, the transmission of genes from generation to generation – but today, we have to think of the transmission, to the following generations, of epigenetic factors – the effect of the phenomenon of gene expression, the transmission of required traits – that is what is called "soft inheritance". We have good reason to anticipate the transformation of Homo sapiens in relation to how we are born. In fact, this is the topic of my book. If you Google the topic, none of them consider the effects of how babies are born – never, never, never! They look at all other possible factors, not realizing that this is the formative phase of human life.

AGB: What do you see as being responsible for the situation?

MO: It's cultural.

AGB: One of the problems could be the tremendous fear of childbirth in women – a primal terror that leads to surgical intervention, whether planned or otherwise.

MO: This fear is not new; that has been the case through the ages. Women were dying!

AGB: Pharmaceutical companies take advantage of this fear – they make billions from fear every year – fear of sadness, fear of pain – without consideration of the social consequences. And the medical industry is much the same.

MO: Always the same way of thinking. In other societies, before the age of industrialization, traditional midwives were giving herbs to relieve the pain, to facilitate labour. It's the same way of thinking as now. It's just that we have more powerful ways in terms of pharmacological assistance. What is not understood is that there has always been a fear of birth, but that nature has a solution to eliminate cultural conditioning during the birth process. The solution is to eliminate the activity of the neocortex [the most recently developed part of the brain]. To protect the labouring woman from any stimulation of the neocortex. The key word is protection. You cannot help, you cannot guide, you cannot control, you cannot support, but you can protect a labouring woman from neocortical stimulation. That is why I often describe a situation as compatible with the easiest birth possible: a woman giving birth with nobody around other than an experienced, silent midwife who sits in a corner, knitting. The absence of neocortical stimulation means that the labouring woman can behave like a mammal. And yet this situation – incredibly simple, unknown in our society – is almost culturally unacceptable! The problem today is not the medicalization of childbirth; it is the socialization of childbirth. The new paradigm would be to learn things from the physiological perspective. The natural childbirth people believe in coaching – the same way of thinking as labour management in medieval circles.

AGB: But what happens when there's a problem with the birth? How can neocortical stimulation be avoided?

MO: The priority in terms of security is to make the birth easy, because an easy birth is less dangerous than a difficult birth. And yet it's not an easy concept for us to understand. We have to start with the understanding that an easy birth is safer than a difficult birth. Having said that, if things aren't going well, there is one alternative: an in-labour, non-emergency caesarean section.

AGB: I was fascinated to read about an experiment with mice who lack the gene responsible for the production of another one of the love hormones. These mice leave their babies unwashed, unfed, unloved. It reminded me of all the stories you read of mothers who viciously abuse or neglect their children – it's as if they're wired incorrectly. In such cases, love is absent.

MO: That is what we have to consider when we address the future of humankind. We can imagine a human being of the future with perhaps a higher degree of encephalisation, perhaps a higher intelligence quotient, but at the same time, dysregulation of the emotional system. There is already a model in that direction: the "Aspies" – the people who have Asperger's syndrome.

AGB: Let me read you a quote from Richard W Tsien, a professor of neuroscience: "Oxytocin has a remarkable effect on the passage of information through the brain. It not only quiets background activity, but also increases the accuracy of stimulated impulse-firing. Our experiments show how the activity of brain circuits can be sharpened, and hint at how this re-tuning of brain circuits might go awry in conditions like autism ... It's too early to say how the lack of oxytocin signalling is involved in the wide diversity of autism-spectrum disorders, and the jury is still out about its possible therapeutic effects. But it is encouraging to find that a naturally occurring neurohormone can enhance brain circuits by dialling up wanted signals while quieting background noise."

MO: Already, there are more and more people with Asperger's. An interesting point: many Nobel prize winners are Aspies – they have very, very high IQs, but cannot understand emotion, they cannot read emotion.

AGB: So how do we ensure that love survives?

MO: That's a good question. Today, if we really want love to survive, we have to flirt with utopia: we have to get out of political correctness. An important point to make is this: to be an obstetrician or to be a midwife, the prerequisite would be to be a mother who had a positive experience of the birth of her babies. It's utopian, and culturally unacceptable. But I am pretty sure that if such a simple rule were introduced, that would be a way to break a vicious cycle. Today it's commonplace to say: we must reduce the rate of caesarean sections. If you say that, everyone agrees. But if you want to introduce a radical way to open a new era, a new phase, you have to be utopian. But today it's culturally unacceptable to suggest ways to make a birth as easy as possible. Immediately, people see obstacles – it's impossible! It's culturally unacceptable! But utopian does not mean impossible.

AGB: The problem is that we don't perceive ourselves as mammals. Such a perspective flies in the face of our conditioning. We perceive ourselves as superior to animals, so your approach calls everything – our values, our priorities – into play. It's a perceptual issue.

MO: In matters of birth, the mother will know what to do if there is nobody else around apart from the midwife. It's not a question of knowledge or experience; it's a question of mammalian instinct.

AGB: Your criteria for the selection of obstetricians and midwives will create great controversy.

MO: Yes. At the present time, people are talking about the education of obstetricians and midwives. I think that's a secondary issue. The primary issue is the selection process. After several generations of medicalized birth, there are not many women who have the ideal personality to be midwives. And when a woman has a positive experience of childbirth – because it's not common – her duty would be to become a midwife! [laughs]

AGB: I still think that women need to be empowered in terms of thinking themselves capable of birthing a child, even if it's only through the assurance that their bodies will simply know how to do it.

MO: For a pregnant woman to meet with women who have enjoyed birth: that is the best kind of education. This was my observation in our maternity unit. We had singing sessions for pregnant women. Young mothers who had given birth and were still in the neonatal unit were coming to the singing group as well, because they could talk together. That was a good education. But I don't think the focus should be on preparation; it's much more to focus on the environment at birth. That is the important point, yes? That way we rectify all the mistakes of the natural childbirth groups that have associated birth preparation with natural childbirth. When the birth is prepared, it's not natural, you see? So we have to be radical. If not, it is useless!

AGB: How can those of us who were birthed in a stressful environment – or those of us who gave birth in a stressful environment – reconnect with our instincts, with our truest feelings? Because it's a far broader issue than birth politics. So many of us live at a distance from ourselves.

MO: The real question is how do we participate in the initiation of this necessary new awareness? We have work at the cultural level. Those who want to share their degree of awareness, those who want to share their intuition, those who want to participate in the initiation of a necessary new awareness must train themselves to be bilingual. What does it mean to be bilingual? It means that if you only use the language of the heart – and natural childbirth groups only use the language of the heart – you are absolutely useless. Today, to be useful, you have to combine this language of the heart with scientific language. The only way to reverse a thousand years of cultural conditioning is to use a scientific language; there is no other way at this present time. The cultural conditioning is too strong. When I was a medical student in 1953 – that is to say, exactly sixty years ago – I spent six months in the maternity unit of a Paris hospital as an externe, a word that means medical student with limited minor responsibilities. At the time, I had never heard of a mother who, after giving birth, said, "Can I keep my baby close to my body?" Never! Never! Never! They were convinced that it was urgent for the midwife to cut the umbilical cord, and to give the baby to somebody who would take care of him or her. At that time in the neonatal unit, babies were kept in the nursery. Mothers were elsewhere. Nobody thought that they should be in the same room. And that was the result of years of conditioning, during which mothers were separated from babies. And then science recognized that a newborn baby needs its mother. Scientists started to look at bonding and colostrum, they looked at the bacteriological, immunological and hormonal perspectives and suddenly we learn that a newborn baby needs its mother. So we need the scientific discipline!

AGB: Why have we become so dependent on scientific ratification?

MO: Because cultural conditioning is strong. It is thousands of years old! And even today when we know rationally that a newborn baby needs its mother, in reality, we always find excuses to separate mothers and newborn babies, to interfere. That's why, in spite of what we can learn from the scientific perspective, it's incredibly difficult to accept situations that can make a birth easy.

AGB: Part of the problem is our perception of equality. Inexplicably, we have come to understand equal as meaning indistinguishable rather than of equal value. Gender has become a political hot potato. It is now verboten to suggest that gender, far from being mutable, is an ancient code, replete with meaning. An ancient duty. The issue of equal rights – the principle of which is, of course, incontestable – has no place in the birthing room; that is, as you say, the domain of women.

MO: It is a difficult issue.

AGB: So why are we so frightened of love?

MO: Because it's the basis of our society! Since the Neolithic revolution, when our ancestors started to domesticate plants and animals, when they started to introduce agriculture and animal husbandry, the basis of our strategy for survival – the strategy used by all human groups – was to dominate nature, and for one human group to dominate others. New concepts of territory! New reasons for conflicts! The only groups who could survive were those who could double up the human potential for aggression. So for thousands of years, the strategy for survival has been domination. And the best way to double up the human potential for aggression is to moderate the capacity for love. To double up the capacity to destroy life, one must interfere at the critical period, the period surrounding birth. Which is how we can explain beliefs such as colostrum is dangerous, mothers must not look into a baby's eyes, there must be no skin-to-skin contact, and so on.

AGB: Which is also how the corporate world justifies the dog-eat-dog philosophy.

MO: Until now, we have only been concerned with the survival of our own human group, but today, suddenly, it's becoming different. The point is not the survival of your human group or my human group, but the survival of humanity. It's new, absolutely. It's new. Today we know there are limits to the domination of nature because we have reached the limit. Today, suddenly, humanity as a whole needs a new strategy for survival. What we need in the future is the energies of love – the capacity to love: love of nature, love of Mother Earth. It was an advantage until now to moderate love for Mother Earth, but today it is complicated. Suddenly, all these beliefs and all these rituals are losing their evolutionary advantage. There is no evolutionary advantage now to say that colostrum is dangerous for the baby. The science says it's precious; we have to listen to science now. Only the scientific perspective has the power to reverse thousands of years of conditioning.

AGB: What happens exactly when mother and baby are separated immediately after birth?

MO: Many things. The newborn baby needs its mother and, at the same time, the mother needs her baby. If the mother is in an ideal situation just after giving birth, she can release a vital high peak of oxytocin – vital because it is necessary for a safe delivery of the placenta and also because oxytocin is the main component of the cocktail of love hormones a woman is supposed to release at that time. To release this high peak of oxytocin the mother must not be distracted. She needs, ideally, to feel the contact with the baby's skin, to look into the baby's eye, and to smell its odour. It is an interaction between mother and newborn baby. For thousands of years, this has not been understood: there has been routine separation between mother and newborn baby. This is a way to explain the high incidence of haemorrhage and the high incidence of maternal deaths, particularly in some cultural milieus.

AGB: You talk a lot about the need for privacy in birth; for the child to be born in privacy. Curiously, there have been corresponding studies that address the moment of death. People often wait until they're left alone to die.

MO: Ah! You speak about being alone – privacy and alone are not the same. Privacy is not feeling observed. In London, for example, in the Tube between Oxford Circus and Victoria Station, you have privacy; you don't feel observed because you are anonymous. But you are not alone. So that's why I never use the term "alone". I talk about not feeling observed, which is different –

AGB: Because a sense of being observed triggers neocortical activity?

MO: When you feel observed, you observe yourself; you activate your neocortex. When mammals feel observed, they increase their level of adrenaline.

AGB: And adrenaline stops the production of oxytocin, which halts the birth?

MO: All mammals have a need not to feel observed while giving birth; it's a basic need.

AGB: So describe a mother's ideal discovery of her baby.

MO: If the mother had a real foetus ejection reflex – something that is almost unknown in our society, but which would be the prototype-kind of undisturbed birth – she would be still in a hormonal flood, a bit on another planet. The mother would look at the baby first, and then become more audacious – touch the baby's body with their fingertips, hold the baby, and most mothers at that point look at the baby's eyes. And it seems that deep eye-to-eye contact is an important phase at the beginning of the mother–baby relationship. One woman told me, "I looked into my baby's eyes and saw the whole universe!" Women have so many ways to describe that first moment.

AGB: You often speak of the "ancient messages". What are these ancient messages that science decodes?

MO: If you read Genesis in the Bible, you read about Eve consuming the fruit of the Tree of Knowledge. You understand through this story the handicap of seeing too much, of knowing too much. And on the same page, you read that because this fruit was eaten, human beings are condemned to have difficult births. This is an example of an old message that has been interpreted through the scientific perspective today: the concept of neocortical inhibition.

AGB: So according to you, the more intelligent the woman, the more complications she is likely to endure when birthing her child?

MO: [laughs] It's not so much a question of intelligence as it is of the relationship between the primitive brain and the neocortex. The capacity to reduce neocortical activity is the issue. Again, to use a cultural reference point: the Bible ends on a message of love. In general, when reading a biography of a famous person, you don't read about how they were birthed, but in the case of the man whose mission was to promote love, the way he was born was part of the story – it was part of the story. So if you read in detail, you learn that his mother reduced neocortical activity by giving birth in a stable with other mammals –

AGB: Ah, yes – but the husband was present!

MO: [laughing] Through science, you can interpret these old stories in a completely new way.

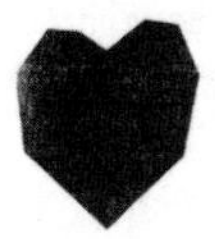

The fairytale ending

Marriage as a mirror

Marriage is not about religion or gender;
it is an admission of vulnerability.

Arriving late at a friend's wedding, I wriggled my way through the crowd to congratulate him and his love. He was busy shaking hands; she had sequestered herself in an alcove with girlfriends. Waving at him over a number of heads, I overheard the new bride say, "I've got it!" Turning, I saw her, resplendent in satins and showcasing – in the manner of a hunter brandishing a carcass – the golden band. Her expression was one of vindication.

This perception of marriage as a victory was alien to me. The first child of a union so oppressive that I left home at sixteen, I had come to regard marriage as a kind of lined box in which women were kept. Yes, I had been conditioned by the same fairytales and their perversely truncated view of a woman's life – one that ends at, or just after, her wedding – but I had also seen what can happen after a wedding. I had studied the photograph album in which my mother – a slice of heavily iced cake – stiffly smiled, and my father, paradoxically, looked radiant; I had watched the black and white footage of the ceremony (all that could be heard during showings was the click of the Super-8 machine and my mother noting, "I didn't know anybody there"); I had also endured the reality of their marriage. Love, I decided, was safe only when experienced at a distance.

In terms of suffering, my experience was not unusual. The latter half of the twentieth century changed the landscape of marriage forever. Contraception, ease of travel, the domestic incorporation of screen-based technologies (television, computers), implementation of no-fault divorces, mood stabilizers and the proliferation of cyberporn were some of the factors that altered people's expectations of each other and themselves.

In the concomitant turbulence, the communities that had buoyed marriages in times of difficulty fractured. Women who had once formed supportive social networks to help each other with their children and the aged were now in offices for most of the day; through necessity, their children were enrolled in daycare and the aged placed in homes. Historically, it was a time of transition, when life stages became demarcated by their environs: daycare, school, university, work, care facility. The sense of liberation was matched only by the growing sense of alienation. Priorities had, almost imperceptibly, shifted from the human to the material.

All around me, marriages were swelling and disintegrating, like paper in water.

My generation was, in effect, the product of a social experiment. If we did not understand marital intimacy, it was because we had not seen it modelled. We lurched from relationship to relationship, dazzled by the newness of meaninglessness, relentless in our search for something even the most perceptive of us could not identify. Yet we were still susceptible to fairytales, as illustrated by the fact that I was thrice engaged before the age of twenty-four. My first two engagements were refuges from an unmanageable family situation. The third was love: I may have been the one to leave, but he broke my heart.

When I remember him, I know I dodged a bullet; I have seen such marriages played out over the years. And yet there was in me a war: I wanted the fairytale, but did not believe that it was possible. My husband's sincerity swayed me. We were married by a Burmese monk on a humid, beautiful afternoon in a rose garden, and waltzed on petals – I wore loose ecru silk and beaded champagne satin mules – to the music of the 1920s.

Our marriage unfolded as many marriages unfold. We were ridiculous – bursting into tears when the other was out for too long, sighing with longing at the sight of each other – but certain difficulties were beginning to establish themselves.

Neither family was happy about the marriage; both had distinct ideas about the sort of partners we should have, and how our lives should then evolve. The pressures applied were unsubtle. (Years later, my husband and I felt we had no choice but to apply for a restraining order against a member of his extended family.) The situation was Shakespearean, but also farcical.

And then life became frightening. The global financial crisis hit. I was nursing our infant daughter at the time, and we were – unknowingly – living in a "sick" building, one riddled with structural problems and toxic mould. Two companies for which my husband worked folded unexpectedly owing him tens of thousands of dollars that we could not afford to lose. Rates across our industry froze. My husband, stunned, found himself out of work. I watched his depression compound. The romance of early parenting had been replaced with a fusion of love – our daughter was irrepressibly joyous – and terror.

She and I started having severe respiratory problems, but despite repeated visits to doctors and to the hospital, no-one could explain it. I hacked through the night for weeks, for months, my little child coughing beside me; my husband was forced to sleep in the other room. We lived in one of the world's most privileged areas, and were slowly being poisoned by our home. Exhausted and terrified, my husband and I began to fight.

Marriage, I thought but did not say, had begun to feel like a noose.

My father was paralyzed by a stroke and, after six months of minor strokes, died. The estate, he had assured me, ran into millions; I received nothing. My husband's grandmother, to whom he had once been close, died a fortnight later. He, too, received nothing from her estate. We were unmanageably in debt. My husband, seeking escape from his frustration and debilitating feelings of failure, retreated into himself. Late at night, when our daughter was asleep, we would hiss at each other like cats. Some of the arguments were merciless. Enraged, I once threw a cup of hot tea at him; he ducked.

The realisation that life would be less complicated if we were single was unspoken. On more occasions than I can remember, I considered leaving my husband: the prospect glowed, a ring I sometimes took out and admired on my hand. But I was chastened by the fact that we had made a promise, not just to one other but to ourselves. Respect, to me, had always been far more significant than marital longevity, and that incorporated respecting my desire for a harmonious union and the compromises therein, for I had been unmarried by choice for a long, long time, and I liked marriage better.

There was also the awareness that we were part of something greater than ourselves. Those who say marriage is no different to cohabitation are perhaps less sensitive to issues of continuity. Legally and socially, marriage provided us with an framework, struts: as a tradition, it predates history. And yet it is still trivialized as no more than "a piece of paper", or by the perception of it as a kind of country club from which those demarcated as undesirable are excluded. But marriage is not about religion or gender; it is an admission of vulnerability, a commitment to the perpetual evaluation of priorities and a social stabilizer. To paraphrase Bette Davis, it ain't no place for sissies.

The fact that marriage survived the twentieth century at all is a testament to faith – in ourselves, in others, and in the relevance of devotion. For in the end, every marriage stands or falls on the capacity for devotion. And it is hard, in a culture that prizes mutability on all levels, to remain dedicated to an ideal that is so often devoid of spontaneity or glamour. There are days when I would happily trade my husband for an Alexander McQueen box clutch. And then there are days I think of him as my witness, my partner, the door to joy. Marriage is never static. There are peaks and troughs, and cycles. It is easy to forget that this shifting landscape is really only ever a reflection of the self. Our capacity for attachment determines the kind of mate we attract, and it is through this mate that we are forever transformed – marriage as alchemy, but also as a mirror.

Far from threatening the institution, de facto relationships only increase its value, allowing relationships to be tested for soundness without the pressure of expectation and providing those who, because of uncertainty, philosophy or unresolved grief, reject the formalization of love. The degree of expense and consideration necessary for the multi-tiered process of marriage, too, increases its value, as does the expensive and multi-tiered process of divorce. Both act as deterrents to the casual dissolution of relationships that may have otherwise survived. The two improvident divorces I have known involved mental illness; the others were the result of reflection, never gratuitously undertaken.

By concluding with a wedding, the fairytales of our childhood convey the impression that the travails of life are behind us once we marry when, in many cases, they have just begun. Fairytales were written in a time of marked gender inequality, when marriage was, for the majority of women, not just advisable but essential for survival. Cinderella, Sleeping Beauty, Snow White, Beauty and the heroines of Charles Perrault, the Brothers Grimm and other folklorists were once vehicles for empowerment and hope, for it was only through a wedding that a woman could be assured a degree of security and status. To be unmarried was to be vulnerable to ridicule, exploitation and poverty, to be damned as a whore or as hopelessly unloved. Our culture has, in this respect, evolved.

In the developed world, utilitarian marriage is an anachronism. Women no longer need to marry for money or for status, but we continue to marry because the fairytale ending has always signified so much more than an ecclesiastical or social rite. A wedding remains the universal symbol of union – the bringing together of two halves, both in the literal sense and in the metaphysical: the beginning of a new journey as an integrated whole. Through fairytales, we are made to understand that all our fractures can be healed.

I no longer perceive marriage as a box. After almost a decade with my husband, I can say that marriage has made me a better human being. Although I still do not perceive my wedding as a victory in terms of a campaign, I do see it as a victory over a romantic impulsivity fuelled by terror. Marriage has calmed me, and shown me the purpose of patience. While I cannot say whether mine will be concluded by biology or design, I do know I'll never regret it, for it is through marriage that I have overcome my fear of love.

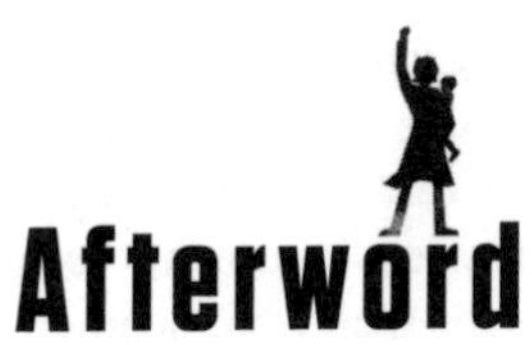

Afterword

Decree Absolute

But this time was different.
This time he left.

My husband left me in the thick of the first wave of publicity for this, a book about my love for him and the child we made together. The irony was not lost on me. He flew almost a thousand kilometres away and made his new home there, in a graceful apartment across the water from his mother's house. We separated two months later. To be fair, he had implored me to join him and I had refused. Proximity to his mother was fourth last on my list of things to do, just before shaving my head with a piece of tin, genocide and DIY infibulation. Still, the quietness of the fracture took me by surprise. No-one yelled. There were no clothes strewn on the driveway. He drank too much one night and became disorientated in the central business district, but that was about it. We had bickered beforehand, yes, but that was nothing new; we had bickered about the same issues for years – namely, his family and my unwillingness to relocate to the city in which they lived.

But this time was different. This time he left.

There were ideological differences between us, certainly. The birth of our daughter Bethesda changed us both in different ways. My love for her was immediate and overwhelming, whereas the expression or experience of his could be hindered by fear. In a moving piece about Bethesda's first few months, he wrote of me: "[T]here she was, rearranging her entire life so as to care for this little person that we had made together, and I didn't seem to give the baby a moment's notice. I just wasn't present. It didn't help, I suppose, that I was the child of divorce at a very young age, and so never had much in the way of a paternal role model. In fact, if anything, I saw the roles of mother and father as completely separate, with the father being the significantly less important entity. So I withdrew – confused and resentful that what seemed so easy to my wife was so difficult for me."

My husband would later recognize the loss in this confusion, and mourn it. He had not had a happy childhood. As Gabor Maté notes of the early lives of those uncomfortable with love, "what should have happened didn't happen." And my husband struggled terribly with his memories. Despite this, we shared so much and for so long. We made such an effort to face each other, and to overcome the complicated legacies of our families.

I had never been so happy. Loving him was as easy as falling off a chair, and I felt like Krishna's mother when our daughter opened her mouth to cry: all the universe sparkled therein.

A friend noted that women pay a high price for writing, and she may be right. I returned to my books when Bethesda started school. My husband had, I think, felt enfolded by my devotion to family, but despite the fact that this devotion remained unflagging, despite the fact that I still worked from home, the shift in focus changed his perception of me and, concomitantly, of himself. In combination with the complexities of his family, this shift fast-tracked the end of our marriage.

It was suggested by a number of friends that my husband, significantly younger and a frustrated artist in a different sphere, felt threatened by the seriousness with which I write books, and also by my established identity as a writer. He may disagree with this, I do not know. What I do know is that he never read a manuscript or showed anything but the most cursory interest in the architecture of my work, and I accepted his indifference, figuring that maybe it was not so important in the final wash. To me, our shared interest in Bethesda trumped all other considerations.

That which I had not considered was the role of a book in both defining and altering consciousness, and *Mama* changed me in ways I had not even thought possible, introducing – and, in one case, returning – me to people whose wisdom would change my life. My husband played no part in this evolution, and I remember one day feeling as if we were standing on an ice floe which was gradually cracking in two. The sense of impotence that accompanied this understanding was heartbreaking, but I could not make him want the same things that I wanted, and nor did I want to.

We separated a fortnight before the ten-year anniversary of our first kiss. He suggested it, and I immediately agreed. There was a tragic clarity to my assent – tragic because our daughter would never know her parents together again – and also a flooding sense of relief, not because I did not love him, but because I no longer felt loved by him, not really. I knew that he had once loved me deeply, and also that that love had been irreversibly battered by circumstance.

The Global Financial Crisis had ruined him financially, sending us into a tailspin. I was ill for almost a year (I am asthmatic, and my health has never been strong), and there had been chaotic situations in both families – deaths, duplicity in relation to an inheritance, multiple relocations, professional setbacks, and the spectacularly obsessive determination of my husband's mother in particular to destroy our marriage (my own mother's indifference to it was a statement in itself).

The fact that my husband eventually buckled to these forces was not evidence of weakness, but of the necessity for us to continue our respective journeys separately. It took me time to digest this truth; I was ill for almost eight weeks straight after our marriage ended, developing, for the first time, a case of erythema multiforme, a rare and unsightly skin disease, and then Bethesda and I were sidelined by a violent two-week episode of 'flu. During that terrible fortnight, she crawled into my bed at three or four in the morning. We were both stupefied by fever; my throat was so swollen that I could only croak. I pushed her away, unable to tolerate the heat of her body or the pain of physical contact. She began to sob without inhibition at this rejection and I began to sob with her.

The night around us, still and clear, contained us as completely as a song.

I told almost no-one about the separation. It all seemed so unreal. I quietly continued homeschooling Bethesda. In the evenings, I swept leaves from the garden as the sea susurrated in the distance. It was only when Bethesda slept that I allowed myself to experience the shock of my new reality. I would lie in bed, staring at the ceiling and feeling nothing - not fear, not hope, not pain, not sadness. The immensity of the future had asserted itself. I had no idea what to think or to expect.

It was during one of those nights – in retrospect, they almost feel wooden - that I acknowledged my husband's role in my life. He had, without consciousness or design, changed me for the better. Through our relationship, I learned tolerance – not only of his weaknesses, but of my own. I learned what it is to endure simultaneous external difficulties in tandem. And, importantly, I learned what it is to deepen intimacy over time. I would have liked to know what it is to deepen intimacy over decades, but this was not my destiny.

Given this, I was determined to find a new model of separation, one based on the respect I felt for my husband's role in my life. "We were friends before we married and we can be friends again," I told him. Repeatedly, I extended my hand to his, seeking accord in our loss. My husband not only turned away, but became addicted to disparagement. His rage at me was blind, mindless. In his grief, he began to lash out in ways that literally stunned me. I struggled to comprehend his rationale, and continued – with increasing desperation – to try to make him see the wisdom of harmony between us. He would not hear. All that mattered to him, he said, were what he understood as his "rights". ("Rights," as a therapist of my acquaintance noted, "are the language of anger.")

And then my husband called in lawyers, and everything that had been good between us unravelled like a spool of thread down stairs, never again to be wound in the same way.

The tenderness I felt for him was, lawyers made clear, not only superfluous but unseemly. "Stop calling him your husband!" my lawyer tersely instructed. What she really wanted was for me to regard him as no more an an obstacle or difficulty I had to overcome. The love I felt for him was a relic; from hereon, he was to be reduced to two clinical words: "the father". This made it clear that my husband's relationship to me was no longer direct, but exclusively through our child. The weight of this role, that of the axis or conduit, sat badly with Bethesda, and I wondered at its impact on any child. Why should children bear the weight of justifying a relationship between two adults? Why does the law not recognize the significance of – and, more importantly, insist on – direct parental affection, respect and civility (outside the parameters of marital and familial abuse)? How is it that parental quarrels are dismissed as irrelevant in relation to children? And, critically, what kind of example do we set our children when we jettison our partners without acknowledgment of the impact of their role in our lives, and without consideration of, or for, their dignity? Because without that, we teach our children that dignity is only to be accorded to those who serve our purposes.

The lawyers' reactions to any proprietorial display on my behalf toward my husband made it clear that attachment is, in this culture, regarded as an indulgence. Were separating couples to be addressed as affective beings with a need for attachment – rather than being reduced to reproductive units – the entire legal framework would have to be revised.

My issue, then, was not, as lawyers presupposed, one of frustrated longing (I did not and do not want my husband back), but of being forced into an artificially dispassionate position. Why should I feign indifference to the man who had fathered my child, and for whose benefit? Not my daughter's, that was for certain. My husband, the child of a drawn-out, "dirty" divorce, delighted in emphasizing the lack of connection between us, but this was only a tantrum; in time, he would have cause for reflection and regret.

Our daughter, shocked by his behaviour toward her and toward me, no longer wanted to speak with him; the space between them soon was an abyss. "Men are disloyal," she told me one night, a statement that filled me with despair. It was easier for my husband to blame me for her anger, too.

I changed our telephone number, and called in a psychologist for Bethesda, whose levels of anger and anxiety were becoming problematic. I focused all my energies on maintaining domestic stability, having taken over the running of the household and homeschooling single-handed, under what sometimes felt like a siege of ugliness. There was no time to process the fact that my marriage had ended – there was no time to process anything.

For six months, I lived in a state of emergency.

Repeatedly, I received instruction on the new worthlessness of mothers from lawyers. My evaluation of my daughter's behaviour was considered irrelevant without the "expert" opinion of a mental health professional. Despite the fact that I am the global authority on my daughter – after giving birth to, five years of cosleeping with, eight years of fulltime care for, and over a year of homeschooling her, there is almost nothing about Bethesda I do not know – my interpretation of her behaviour was dismissed with the same patronising degree of scepticism and prejudice shown to women in the Victorian era. The responses reminded me of the nineteenth century criminologist Cesare Lombroso's quote: "Women have many traits in common with children; that their moral sense is deficient; that they are revengeful, jealous, inclined to vengeances of a refined cruelty."

When I told lawyers that my daughter was seriously traumatised, it was, in effect, meaningless; their view was a gender reversal of Mandy Rice-Davies' damning assessment of Viscount Astor ("Well, she would say that, wouldn't she?"). My motherhood immediately made me suspect: without any evidence, I was presumed vengeful, irrational, jealous, inclined to cruelty. However, if a psychologist who knew nothing of the family situation came to the same conclusion about my daughter's behaviour after six forty-minute sessions, it would be considered a significant statement.

I met a beautiful pregnant woman who preferred being rendered homeless than to have the father of her unborn child pay maintenance as she was terrified that he would then assert his "rights"; I met a documentary maker who battled the violent father of her child in court to stop him having access to their child (again, his "right"). One professionally successful mother, in a desperate effort to protect her children from her husband's drug use, consulted a child psychologist who said, "Assuming you're not making it up, your partner's drug use doesn't interest me. I'm not here to take sides." I had women helplessly sobbing in my arms at bookshop talks as they recounted what had happened to them after separation. In time, two things became clear (and I refer to normal situations): mothers are no longer permitted the tender sense of guardianship over babies that constitutes the bedrock of maternal-infant attachment, and fathers no longer feel they are required to treat the mothers of their children with respect.

Incredibly, both situations are facilitated and protected by the law.

A social worker to whom I spoke elaborated. "We live in a patriarchal society, and this is reflected in family law. Mothers are now seen as irrelevant or as interchangeable with any other carer. The system used to be loaded against fathers, and now it's the opposite. Complaints by mothers, no matter how justified, are reframed as the ravings of a vindictive wife. I cannot tell you the cases I have dealt with that defy description – wife-beaters who end up with custody of the children, who then end up in care when they are found to have been beaten by the father; children who end up in the care of paedophiles; children who end up with unbelievable psychological damage as a result of the wars created by angry fathers. It has taken the deaths of countless children to wake people up. The system is only beginning to change now, but slowly. It is a disgrace."

Throughout the separation, I struggled to remain centred, not only for Bethesda's sake but for my own. I made a promise to remember why I had chosen to marry my husband. Easier said. The way he behaved in the wake of our split made me understand for the first time why some women cut their husband's faces out of wedding photographs. At one point, I was tempted to auction my wedding band on eBay, but realized that the ring would have significance for Bethesda, whom I did not want to grow up thinking that I had never loved her father. I recognized that my impulse had been spiteful and petty, and that such responses had no place in my life. It was time to grow up.

One afternoon, Bethesda, who had been difficult for weeks, suddenly screamed, "*Why is this happening to us?! Why??*" This last word echoed until it assumed an almost physical presence. Without hesitating, I enfolded her in my arms. "Why not?" I softly replied. My answer startled her, but then she got it: devastation isn't personal. It happens to everyone, every day, everywhere.

Who were we to be exempt from pain?

Having survived my 32-year-old brother's suicide, I was not destroyed by the end of my marriage. I may have failed in my efforts to create a loving separation, but there is this: no-one is ill, no-one has died. Bethesda still raises her arms to me, wanting an embrace. Our cat still bumps his forehead to mine. I am still here. Melodrama is of no interest. I know that I will not only passionately love again, but that I will again feel carelessly happy. This is the nature of existence. Joy always returns.

Inevitably, I sometimes miss being married. I do not miss my husband as he is, but as he was. He will exist forever in my memory as a young father standing on a high green hill in the sunshine, throwing our laughing three-year-old daughter in the air as far behind us, a wedding party hoots and cheers at the bride, a dear friend. Even now, my eyes fill as I write these words, remembering.

The fact that my husband did not fulfill my fantasies or expectations does not preclude my caring for him. And how could I not care? He is the father of my only child; I will never give birth to another. Without him, Bethesda would not exist and I would never have experienced the rich and wild and textured intimacy we shared. In denying his impact on my life, I would be suppressing truth and in that, holding onto him. Instead, I let my husband go and with him, my every heartfelt blessing. Goodbye, Alex. I will always be so grateful that I fell in love with him and he with me.

My former mother-in-law is, of course, a different story.

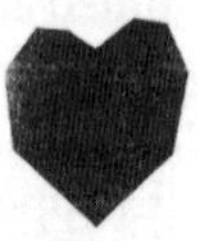

ANTONELLA GAMBOTTO-BURKE'S RECOMMENDED BOOKS

For every child:

Charlotte's Web EB White, illustrated by Garth Williams
Half Magic Edward Eager, illustrated by NM Bodecker
The Phantom Tollbooth Norton Juster, illustrated by Jules Feiffer
Good Night, Fairies Kathleen Hague, illustrated by Michael Hague
Show Me How to Survive Joseph Pred
A Book of Spooks and Spectres Ruth Manning Sanders, illustrated by Robin Jacques
Harry Potter and the Philosopher's Stone JK Rowling, illustrated by Mary GrandPré
The Folk of the Faraway Tree Enid Blyton
Cole's Funny Picture Book #1 Edward Cole
The Random House Children's Treasure Chest edited by Alice Mills

For every parent:

What Every Parent Needs to Know: The Incredible Effects of Love, Nurture and Play on Your Child's Development Margot Sunderland

Peaceful Parent, Happy Kids: How to Stop Yelling and Start Connecting Laura Markham

Transforming the Difficult Child: The Nurtured Heart Approach Howard Glasser and Jennifer Easley

Thou Shalt Not Be Aware: Society's Betrayal of the Child Alice Miller

The NDD Book: How Nutrition Deficit Disorder Affects Your Child's Learning, Behaviour, and Health, and What You Can Do About It – Without Drugs William Sears

Raising Babies: Why Your Love is Best Steve Biddulph

Hold on to Your Kids: Why Parents Need to Matter More than Peers Gordon Neufeld and Gabor Maté

Attached at the Heart: Eight Proven Parenting Principles for Raising Connected and Compassionate Children Barbara Nicholson and Lysa Parker

The Continuum Concept: In Search of Happiness Lost Jean Liedloff

Primal Health: Understanding the Critical Period Between Conception and the First Birthday by Michel Odent

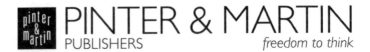

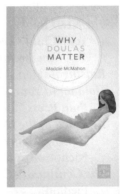

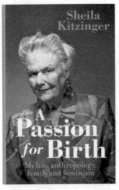

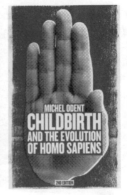

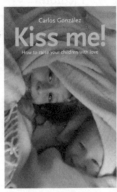

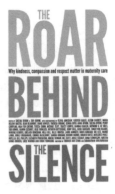

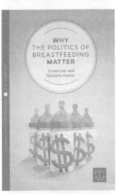

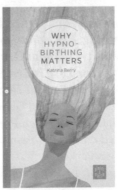

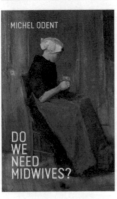

EMBARKING ON
AN ADVENTURE WITH GOD

EMBARKING ON AN ADVENTURE WITH GOD

Finding Spiritual Fulfillment

Dr. Karen M. Jackson

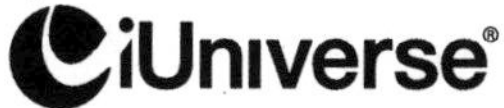

EMBARKING ON AN ADVENTURE WITH GOD
FINDING SPIRITUAL FULFILLMENT

iUniverse books may be ordered through booksellers or by contacting:

iUniverse
1663 Liberty Drive
Bloomington, IN 47403
www.iuniverse.com
1-800-Authors (1-800-288-4677)

ISBN: 978-1-4917-9520-0 (sc)
ISBN: 978-1-4917-9512-5 (e)

Library of Congress Control Number: 2016907038

Print information available on the last page.

iUniverse rev. date: 05/04/2016

TABLE OF CONTENTS

DEDICATION

This book is dedicated to my
Grandmother, Beatrice Chaney Bell
Aunt, Rita Franks-Bell
and
Best friend, Ronnie Alexander Jones.

Although you are gone, I feel your presence every day.
You are and forever will be the source of my determination
in accomplishing my dreams.

INTRODUCTION

Ok, no problem. That was my thinking when my employer handed me a memo to attend a conference for the record. As an administrator I knew when you received a letter like this it couldn't be good news, but surely it would be different for me. After all, I am a child of God. All I had to do was put everything in place I had been taught as a Christian. Pray, trust, believe, don't doubt, and stand on God's word. What an awesome opportunity to finally use what I've been taught. This was going to be evidence of God working a miracle, and boy, the testimony I was going to share.

Little did I know this life changing event was the start of an adventure I would be embarking on with God. I remember focusing on all the negative aspects of losing my job. I knew I wasn't the first person to have this happen, but I was still angry. I isolated myself from family and friends and wanted revenge on those who had "wronged me". Every day was becoming more confusing to the point I was becoming upset with God. I have my doctorate degree, a wealth of knowledge, many years of experience and friends in "high" places. So, why weren't doors being opened on my behalf? Minister Dr. Karen Jackson was a household name within my community. I had people who looked up to me when it came to my inner strength and resilience in God. I knew and studied the Word and applied it daily. I had the ability to help others overcome their obstacles and make a difference in their lives. Reviewing my life from then to now, I realized I had hit rock bottom, cowering to my lowest emotions. I knew I had to change my perspective from despair, fear, stress, hatred and brokenness to that of joy, excitement, contentment and enthusiasm. It was time to refocus. My attitude about my situation was not getting me anywhere. As a matter of fact, it stunk! I had to finally reassess my life and realize what I was going through was part of a plan God had for me. I had to be a willing vessel and allow God to take control of my life. I did not know what He was doing or where He was leading me, but I did know I had to trust Him. I had to look at it for what it really was an adventure God had specifically chosen for me to embark on with Him.

Jeremiah 29:11 (NLT) states, *"I know the thoughts that I think toward you, saith the Lord, thoughts of peace, and not of evil, to give you an expected end."* There is so much God wants His children to be blessed with, to experience. Yes, we all want to stay with the familiar, but if we do not allow God to "move" us, we will never experience the goodness and mercy only He can provide. God wants to do amazing things in our lives, if only we would be willing to submit to Him. This is why the adventure is so important. God wants us to be blessed with our "expected end."

As you read this book, it is my sincere hope you evaluate what you are currently going through in your life. How you view your current situation, such as the loss of a loved one, health or family issues, stress factors or involvement with other crises, will dictate your adventure. You can't allow your situation to take control and distance you from God.

This book will allow you to explore your true emotions and validate your stance as a child of God. It is ok to experience pain, fear, grief, and anxiety, all of which are natural emotions. You are human. The secret is not to allow these emotions to consume you. You will gain insight when you realize you are exactly where God wants you to be. This is your preparation for greatness.

Life is not always easy, but it is your endurance which will sustain you while on your adventure. It's the willingness to persevere no matter what is blocking your path. By the end of your adventure, your focus will shift to the inner strength you did not know you had! You will come to appreciate the wondrous blessings of God even more. Be willing to embark on the adventure with Him, despite how the situation looks and complete the journey. Your relationship with God will go to a totally different level.

You will witness firsthand the awesomeness of God. Yes, there will be heartaches, pain, and disappointments, but you will also experience the excitement only an adventure with God will give you. Allow God to take hold of you and lead you into the unknown. Make yourself available. Get ready to experience the unexpected.

CHAPTER 1

Embarking on an Adventure with God

Embark – To set out on a venture

Have you ever thought back on the plans you had for your life? Are you happy and content? Do you feel fulfilled or just going through the motions? Now think what would happen if everything changed. How would you handle change? These are the questions which may occur when it seems God is challenging you to evaluate your life. Change occurs when God has a special assignment only you can fulfill. Did your plans include what God wanted for your life? There are instances when God intercedes in your life because it is the perfect opportunity for you to embark on an adventure with him.

1 Samuel tells the story of King David and his humble beginnings. David was a shepherd who tended sheep. He had no other plans beyond that, but God had already predetermined he would be king of Israel. God told Samuel to go visit a man named Jesse, who lives in Bethlehem. *"I've chosen one of his sons to be my king."* (1 Samuel 16). That son was David. One can only imagine how David felt. There he was tending sheep and probably thinking to himself how happy he was with his life. But God had other plans for David, just like He has plans for all His children. There are many stories in the bible where David encounters different obstacles (See chapter 5) before he ultimately becomes King. What a blessing it is to know God has predestined our lives. Take for example the story of Kristina.

It was a season of change for Kristina. She had completed her engineering degree and found a job working with a high profile firm. She had two promotions within six months, a signing bonus and expense account. Kristina traveled all over the world and was climbing her way up the corporate ladder. Overnight, she was out of a job with no explanation. She felt her world had been turned upside down. Kristina chose not to focus on her situation, but to concentrate on God. She knew when God has plans for your life he has to uproot you so those plans can come to fulfillment. Maybe this was her season of rest in preparation for the changes that were soon to take place. It may have been her season of decrease, only to experience the increase God was going to provide. Although she encountered different obstacles, she maintained her relationship with God and he blessed her with a better job. Kristina is engaged and looking forward to raising a God-fearing family. She learned that when you embark on an adventure with God, you have to:

- Be still and listen to God's voice.
- Be a willing vessel.
- Allow God to take total control of your life.
- Be obedient to God's commands.

There are times when God has to take control of your life for your purpose to be fulfilled. Like Kristina, if he hadn't moved on my behalf, I would still be daydreaming in the same spot I was 10 years ago. My assignment was unique and specifically mapped out for me. No one else could travel the road God was taking me on. It is important to totally submit yourself to God and allow him to intercede in your life. Despite your experiences, learn not to give up or lose hope.

Consider the children of Israel who were living in bondage for over 400 years. Although they prayed for deliverance, they had come to accept their situation. Their adventure began when God sent Moses to intercede on their behalf. Pharaoh was hardhearted and refused to release them. Moses was faithful and never wavered in following God's instructions. Finally, after the 10th plague, Pharaoh agreed to release them (Exodus 12:29-31). They had no time to prepare for their journey. An adventure can be so rushed you may not have time to prepare for the journey. God's timing is perfect, which is why you have to always be ready.

When God delivered the children of Israel, they started to complain and grumble because they lost their focus. They fervently asked God to deliver them from bondage. They soon forgot what God had done and the prayers that were answered, mirroring my attitude - bondage. Although it was a familiar bondage, God decided to uproot me. I began to murmur and complain because I didn't like the direction my life was taking. I started to question God. Why is this happening to me? How am I going to survive? How long is this going to take? To me, these were valid questions. I had embarked on an adventure with God and didn't know what to expect. Although I became rebellious, God continued to be faithful.

God is going to supply you with everything you need for your journey. God wants you to totally depend on Him and your adventure will do just that – allow you to become powerless so he can prove to you how powerful He is. When your enemies try to encamp around you, God will open your "Red Sea". This will give you an opportunity to leave your past and enter into the new life God has for you. The key is to remain faithful and steadfast.

When the Israelites were preparing to enter the land God promised them, Moses sent 12 men to explore the land (Numbers 13). The purpose was not to see if they could enter the land, God already promised it to them. The purpose was for them to know what to expect. God is never going to lead you blindly into situations He has already preordained for you. The scouts came back with varying reports. They all agreed the land was plentiful. It was rich with milk and honey. But instead of focusing on all the "positives", ten of the men gave details on the "negatives". *"The people who live there are strong and their cities are large and walled. These people are too much for us"* (Numbers 13:28). This would have been an excellent opportunity for them to focus on the goodness of God. The key is to focus on the positive aspects of your adventure and what God has for you. Because of the Israelites unbelief, God had them wander 40 years. Do you really have that much time to wander because you didn't trust God?

You are going to experience a whirlwind of emotions that will overtake you. You will wonder if you even have the stamina to complete this adventure. At some point you may question God as to why you are going through this. There will be tears. Allow me to encourage you right now. God has placed everything within you to complete this adventure with him. Don't even think about giving up! Your life will change dramatically so you mustn't lose sight.

There are many paths God is going to have you travel. That's what's so awesome about the adventure; every day will bring new and unique experiences. God will place people in your life for a season, some longer than others. Each person will have a different impact on your life. You will travel to places you would have never gone before. Your experiences will enhance your character and your testimony. There is a great blessing waiting for you.

God could have chosen anyone else to embark on this adventure with him, but he chose YOU! He considered you because he has seen your faithfulness. You are blessed and highly favored. You have been set apart for a special purpose which will be revealed to you by the end of your adventure. The pieces will start to come together like a puzzle whose picture is not complete until the final piece is added. God wants to do so much for you. He wants to answer prayers and elevate you to heights you never dreamed of. God will restore everything taken from you. I am a witness he will give you "double for your trouble".

Reflection Questions

1. *Are there issues you are currently facing?*
2. *How has God interceded in your life? Is this your "wake up" call?*
3. *Do you feel God is preparing you for an adventure with him? How has He revealed this to you?*
4. *Describe your emotions regarding your impending adventure with God. Are they valid?*
5. *Keep a diary of your adventure. Use this as a reflection tool to document your emotions.*

CHAPTER 2

The Adventure Begins

Adventure – An unusual or exciting experience

God allows events to happen in our lives to make us "move" to fulfill our destiny. For many, this "movement" is a change of scenery, allowing us to meet new people and take us to places we may have never dreamed of going. Your task is to be obedient and walk the journey God has for you with confidence.

In the book of Ruth we are introduced to two women, Ruth and Naomi, who are embarking on their own adventure with God. Tragedy became the bond that fused them together. Ruth's husband dies and Naomi has previously lost her husband and now, two sons. With the loss of everything, Naomi realizes she has nothing to offer her daughter in laws. She had no relatives in Moab and was not even sure how she was going to be accepted in her homeland, Israel. Naomi wanted Ruth to stay in Moab with her family, but she refused. Although Naomi was going to unfamiliar territory, Ruth was willing to accompany her. Obviously, Ruth saw something in Naomi that made her want to follow her. In fact, she "clung" to Naomi. They had become inseparable and their greatest bond was their faith in God. Ruth tells Naomi, *"Don't ask me to leave you and turn back. Wherever you go, I will go; wherever you live, I will live. Your people will be my people, and your God will be my God."* (Ruth 1:16). Little did Ruth realize the adventure she was about to embark on with Naomi.

In hindsight, it would have been easy for Ruth to return home to her family. Who wouldn't want to go to a place and people who are familiar? To be honest, that's what I wanted. I wanted to go back to my old routine, co-workers, and familiar way of life. I realized through my personal tragedy - the loss of a job, depression, grief and the feeling of loneliness - that I had to gather the courage I needed to forge ahead, refusing to turn back.

When the women go to Bethlehem, Ruth gets busy. She doesn't just sit around feeling sorry for herself. She goes to work in the fields because it is harvest time. Instead of depending on Naomi, she took the first step and went to work. She knew there were needs to be met and God would supply them. While working in the fields, Ruth is noticed as a hard worker. Her qualities enhanced her reputation. Instead of complaining, she chooses to be faithful and brave. She knew wherever God was leading her, she had to be consistent with a positive attitude, despite the circumstances she found herself in. Eventually, she found favor with the field's owner, Boaz, who made sure she was well taken care of.

I remember sitting around the house feeling sorry for myself. I had become an introvert, lost to darkness. It was time for me to take MY first step. While waiting for my circumstance to change, I decided to make a difference in the lives of others. I volunteered for the AIDS Foundation and did it faithfully. As I went about my daily routine, I found myself being applauded for my hard work and dedication. God was working in my life. My reputation was growing. Why? Because I was dedicated to the assignment God had given me. No, it wasn't for money, fame or fortune, but it was for the development of my character. It was part of my adventure!

Eventually, Ruth marries Boaz and their generations include King David and Jesus Christ.

To put it plainly:

- **If there was not a famine, Naomi would not have met Ruth.**
- **If Ruth had not clung to Naomi, she would not have gone to Bethlehem.**
- **If she had not gone to Bethlehem, she would not have started working in the fields.**
- **If she had not worked in the fields, she would have not been noticed by the workers.**
- **If she had not been noticed by the workers, she would have never met Boaz.**

- **If she had not met Boaz, she would have never married him.**
- **If she had not married Boaz, she would not have had a son named Obed, the father of Jesse and the grandfather of Israel's greatest King, David.**

See how it works. You cannot take your adventure lightly. God will take you to unknown destinations and place people in your life for a purpose. The key is to trust the plan He has for you. Now my daily prayer is, "Lord, allow me to travel to these unknown places and meet people who will be a blessing to me." You will never know your "ifs" if you don't take that first step!

Reflection Questions

1. *Have you ever been in a situation where the choice(s) you made was going to change your life dramatically?*
2. *Do you feel comfortable going to unknown places? Why/Why not?*
3. *How do you interact with others?*
4. *What does your character say about you?*
5. *Think of your "ifs". How have they changed your life?*

CHAPTER 3

Fear (Not)

Fear - To feel apprehensive or uneasy

When you embark on an adventure with God, fear is one of the first challenges you will deal with. It is a normal emotion everyone experiences at some point in their life. It paralyzes you, causing uneasiness when you can't see the entire picture. You are presented with circumstances you don't feel you may have the strength to endure, which causes your fear to erupt. Yes, fear is real. My fear began as soon as I received the letter to attend a "Conference for the Record". I kept wondering what it could be about. Why did I receive this letter? Was this a warning? Was I being moved to a different location? Had I done something against company policy? My fear began as the "fear of not knowing". My fear escalated the morning of my conference, even though I had asked God for peace regardless of the outcome. My fear boiled over when I found out I no longer had a job and would have to reapply for another position. Now I was consumed with it! Fear must be confronted and eliminated while you are on your adventure.

The enemy wants you to believe the situation you are going through is catastrophic and you will never recover from it. He doesn't want you embarking on this or any other adventure with God, so he allows fear to block your adventure and ultimately your blessings. We cannot give in to this trickery. You have power through the Holy Spirit to prevail. So the question becomes, "How can I overcome my fears?"

Confront your fears

The Lord is my light and my salvation, so why should I be afraid? (Psalm 27:1).

Fear has the ability to control you if it is not confronted. It keeps you in the background by refusing to allow you to move forward and limiting what you are willing to try. In order to confront your fears, consider the following;

- Talk to a close friend or family member and express your fears.
- If you are worried about your situation, add structure to your life. This will give you a sense of security.
- Assess your spiritual life and seek scriptures which focus on ways to overcome fear. The book of Psalm is an excellent resource.

I allowed fear to dictate my adventure. Despite my faith in God, fear kept telling me, "There is no way your situation is going to change." I had been in my "storm" for so long, everything seemed hopeless. I couldn't feel God's presence and it was bothering me. I had to confront my fear by literally speaking to my situation. I told fear, "I WILL NOT ALLOW YOU CONTROL MY LIFE ANYMORE. EFFECTIVE IMMEDIATELY, I REFUSE TO BE YOUR PRISONER!"

Psalm 27 became my lifeline. I reaffirmed my confidence in God; therefore, I was able to continue my adventure. I no longer carried around excess baggage. I had my control back.

Resist Fear

God has not given us the spirit of fear; but of power, and of love, and of a sound mind. (2 Timothy 1:6-7).

If God has not given us a spirit of fear, why do we feel the need to embrace it? The answer is simple. It exhibits itself based on our past experiences. Think of it as a bad habit. Telling someone to resist it is easier said than done. It takes commitment, but you can break this tendency.

The very moment fear creeps in your spirit – reject it by:

- Focusing on the promises of God. Embrace his blessings.
- Focus on your potential and what God wants you to do.

- Do not allow the enemy to intimidate you. He is the little voice who enters your subconscious and wants you to cower down. This allows him to become the source of your fear.

When the angel of God visited Mary, the mother of Jesus, he told her to fear not because she had found favor with God (Luke 1:26-38). Mary could have chosen to be fearful because:

- She was a virgin who was pregnant.
- She was young and not married. She would become an outcast in her community.
- People (family, friends, and community) would think she was crazy if she tried to explain she had never been with a man.
- Her fiancé could choose not to marry her and have her stoned.

Although Mary was confused she was able to replace her fear with the promise of the Holy Spirit. She received reassurance that with God, nothing was impossible (Luke 1:37). The key to resisting fear is knowing God is in total control. Mary's final response is to acknowledge, *"I am the Lord's servant. May everything you have said about me come true."* (Luke 1:38). When you have acknowledged God and truly submit yourself to Him, you come to realize the plan He has for your life. Remember, God doesn't give his children the spirit of fear. Embrace what He does give: power, love and a sound mind.

Replace Fear with Peace

And the peace of God, which surpasses all understanding, will guard your hearts and minds through Christ Jesus (Philippians 4:7).

Instead of being fearful of things you cannot control, try replacing it with peace. Think about it, you can't do anything about it anyway. God can speak one word commands which can totally change your situation. I knew all God had to say was, "let" and my situation of being unemployed and depressed would change immediately, but God gave me peace.

I surprised myself on how calm I was becoming on my adventure. Instead of continuing to live my life in chaos, I made a conscientious effort to ask God daily for the peace only He could provide. One day my husband came home and told me he had been suspended from his job for 5 days without pay. Before my adventure, I would have panicked, wondering how we were going to make it over this mountain. I was already in a storm and now my husband was joining me. Instead of focusing on the fear stirring inside, I decided to turn it over to God. I was not going to allow anything or anyone to take my peace. It worked! We moved on and didn't even notice the lost wages.

"*The Lord is with me; I will not be afraid.*" (Psalm 118:6) Who better to embark on an adventure with? When you're in the presence of God you are spiritually covered. Think of it this way, God is the captain of your ship. Anchor your trust in Him. God has plenty of experience and has already mapped out your entire adventure. With that being said, why are you still fearful?

Reflection Questions

1. *What fears do you need to conquer?*
2. *What is the source of your fear?*
3. *If God has not given us the spirit of fear, why do you feel so many Christians allow it to interfere with their adventure?*
4. *What causes the "enemy" to intimidate us?*

CHAPTER 4

The Power of Prayer

Prayer – A spiritual communion with God

Prayer is one of the most important things you will need on your adventure. It is the constant communication we have with God – an opportunity for us to pour our heart out and to hear from Him. It is vital to set aside time and pray every day. I remember praying but not really believing God was hearing me. Sure, I said all the right things and even quoted scripture, but my spirit was not lined up with what I was praying to God for. My problem was God did not answer my prayer instantly so I became troubled. I started to believe things were never going to change. It is important to know God's timetable is not yours. Eventually, my prayer life became one of obligation and not sincerity. I found myself going through the motions of prayer but not pausing to hear God's response.

God answers prayers. The problem is it may not be the answer we are expecting. I wanted God to change my situation and the answer was, "No, I have something better for you." A "no" answer does not imply God doesn't care about you or your predicament. God's answer to my request was a wakeup call. It was time for me to stop being spoiled and expecting everything to be given to me instantly. God had an assignment chosen specifically for me and I had to stop being stagnant. It is so important to listen to God's response to our prayers. We need to feel him moving on our behalf, even when we may not agree with His answer.

Pray that God's Will Be Done

*Your **will** be done on earth, as it is in heaven (Matthew 6:10).*

*We continually ask God to fill you with the knowledge of his **will** through all the wisdom and understanding that the Spirit gives (Colossians 1:9.)*

One of the most important prayers you have to keep in the forefront of your mind is to ask God to allow His will to be done. Essentially you are submitting yourself to God and letting Him know you are an available vessel. When I asked God to allow His will to be done in my life, I didn't really realize what I was asking. I wanted HIS will to be done, but on MY terms. I wanted the road to be easy. I didn't expect to lose my job, friends and almost my mind. I didn't want Him to close doors in my life. I didn't want the adventure to last over a year. I didn't want to wake up every morning to a tear stained pillow. Notice the "I's" when I asked God's will to be done. That's the hard part – accepting what He deems best.

I found the closer I became to God, the more I understood the will He had for my life. I totally surrendered to God excited He had revealed my life's purpose. No, it wasn't to tear me down, but to build me up for my life's mission.

Pray for Strength

I can do all things through Christ who strengthens me (Philippians 4:13).

I can't tell you how many times I have heard people recite this verse. The words in this verse never fully materialized until I found myself at my weakest point. Before we get to this key verse, Paul points out something very important. He states, "*I learned*" (Philippians 4:12). To learn something implies you did not have knowledge of it previously. I never knew what it was to be without a hope or future, until the fateful day when everything I had become familiar with was taken from me. I had to learn to be satisfied with where I was in my life; knowing God was going to meet my needs. Yes, I had finally learned something I never knew before – ***I actually could do anything through Christ Jesus who was strengthening me.*** It wasn't money, prestige or a position I could put my trust in. Those things can be taken away in the twinkling of an eye. It was only God who was going to give me the strength I needed. It was this strength that allowed me to continue on my adventure even when things seemed hopeless.

Pray for God's Grace

And he said unto me, My grace is sufficient for thee: for my strength is made perfect in weakness (2 Corinthians 12:9).

Paul had a thorn in his side and he asked God 3 times to remove it. We don't know what Paul's thorn was, but it was significant enough for him to cry out to God. Although God did not remove Paul's affliction, He gave him something even better to deal with it – grace. "*So now I am glad to boast about my weaknesses, so that the power of Christ can work through me. That's why I take pleasure in my weaknesses and in the insults, hardships, persecutions, and troubles that I suffer for Christ. For when I am weak, then I am strong.*" (2 Corinthians 12: 9-10).

I questioned if I had fallen out of God's grace. I prayed daily to God for my ordeal to be over but His answer gave me something amazing that was going to allow me to endure my pain – GRACE. Grace is not earned or deserved. It is given through God's love. I knew it was time for me to apply God's grace to my life and let go of the past. This was the only way I was going to grow spiritually. It was this divine favor that gave me the strength each morning to get up and be excited about the day ahead. I learned to depend less on me and more on God.

Pray for Guidance

Trust in the Lord with all your heart and do not lean on your own understanding. In all your ways acknowledge Him, and He will make your paths straight (Proverbs 3:5-6).

Life's highway can become overwhelming, especially when you aren't sure where God is taking you. Trying to make sense of it will only set you up for an adventure that becomes difficult. Leaning to our understanding only causes fear, anxiety, doubt and confusion. This is not God's intention. He wants to make the path clear of the potholes that can damage your life. The solution is to trust God and pray for guidance. Once you receive your answer, meditate on the Word. Continue to ask for guidance because constant communication is important. Ask God for discernment throughout your adventure to be sure you are following the path He wants you to take.

The enemy will try to come in and convince you to take a different path. In the midst of my adventure, there were times I wanted to go in a different direction. It would have ended my adventure earlier, but deep down inside, it didn't feel right. I prayed and asked God to block any decision or action I wanted to take that was not preordained by Him. My adventure continued. If I did not have a relationship with God through prayer, I would have missed out on the numerous opportunities awaiting me.

Be Persistent in your prayer

So let's not get tired of doing what is good. At just the right time we will reap a harvest of blessing if we don't give up (Galatians 6:9).

No matter how long you have been praying for your situation to change, don't give up! I found myself growing impatient with myself and God. I had to remind myself that God answers prayers according to His timing. Persistence was the key to unlocking the doors I wanted God to open. *"And so I tell you, keep on asking, and you will receive what you ask for. Keep on seeking, and you will find. Keep on knocking, and the door will be opened to you."* (Luke 11:9-10). Your prayers, when aligned to God's will, will not be rejected. Persistence enhances your relationship with God and can bring expected blessings. At God's appointed time, your breakthrough will occur. Be steadfast and firm in your requests, knowing God hears you.

Of course, there is an abundant of prayers which will be utilized. These prayers will be specific to your situation. *"Don't worry about anything; instead, pray about everything; Tell God what you need and thank Him for all he has done. Then you will experience God's peace, which exceeds anything we can understand."* (Philippians 4:6-7). Notice that Paul gives advice to not worry, but pray. Essentially, prayer has to replace any worries you have. The main thing is to pray.

Reflection Questions

1. *How would you describe your prayer life?*
2. *How has God answered your prayers? What was your reaction to His response?*
3. *Do you know God's will for your life?*
4. *How has God strengthened you through prayer?*

CHAPTER 5

Overcoming Obstacles (Giants)

Obstacles (giants) - a thing that blocks one's way or prevents or hinders progress.

As you embark on your adventure with God, you will have to be prepared for the giants you will surely face. When God prepares you for an assignment, any obstacle you confront has been permitted by Him. I know it sounds crazy, but let's examine the facts. God has authority over every area of your life. Nothing can occur unless He allows it. The employer who closed your position, God allowed it. That illness you are experiencing, God allowed it. Why? God is familiar with your resume. He already knows you have everything within yourself to overcome your obstacles.

As mentioned in Chapter 1, David was a man after God's own heart. One would wonder - if David was a man after God's own heart, why did he have to overcome so many obstacles? If we are made in the image of God, why do we have to overcome obstacles? Simply put, this is part of our adventure. Yes, God loves us and we are men and women after God's own heart. Our adventure allows us to be all God wants us to be. He has to prepare all His children for giants so we will know how to overcome them.

David faced a number of giants in his life, the first being Goliath. David's father sends him to take a basket of goods to give to his brothers and their captain who are fighting in Saul's army. At the time, Goliath is taunting the Israeli army. When the army saw the giant, they began to run away in fright. Now, let's not be judgmental of Saul's army. Let's face it, when we encounter giants in our life, our first impulse is to avoid them. Some of the giants you may face include finances, stress, family, depression, grief, and health. David tells Saul not to worry about that Philistine. I'll go fight him (1 Samuel 17:32). Saul gives David an excuse as to why he is no match for Goliath. In your life, there will be people who give you reasons why you can't defeat your giants:

- Age
- Experience
- Education
- Lack of preparation

David gave his reasons that made him qualified to face Goliath. He recounted how he killed a lion and bear who had threatened his family's sheep. He knew the Lord who delivered him from the paw of the lion and from the paw of the bear was going to deliver him from the hand of Goliath (1 Samuel 17:36). As you encounter giants, review your qualifications. Think of a time when you have been victorious over your enemies. Reflect on those things. Those thoughts will reassure you of your capability in defeating your giants. Your response can be the same as David's. "I will go and stand up to them!"

As David prepares to go to battle, Saul gives him his armor to wear. David tried it on, took a step forward and realized he could not go in Saul's armor. As you prepare to fight giants, realize that you cannot use the same weapons that may have been successful for someone else. This goes back to our uniqueness. Everyone's adventure is different, and to try to travel it the same way someone else did is useless. David picked up 5 smooth stones and put them in his shepherd's bag. Armed only with his shepherd's staff and sling, he walked boldly across the valley to Goliath. The lesson is to use what you have at your disposal throughout your adventure.

David not only defeated Goliath, but there were other obstacles he had to overcome:

- Saul's Jealousy (1 Samuel 18)
- The Israelite Army (1 Samuel 30)
- Family (2 Samuel 15-19)
- Self Satisfaction (2 Samuel 11)

The giants you encounter cannot be defeated by your own might. David succeeded in everything he did because the Lord was with him. As you go on your journey, give God the credit He so richly deserves. This is why your enemies are jealous and can't conquer you. They recognize the power of God in your life. You are more than a conqueror.

Reflection Questions

1. *What giants have you encountered while on your adventure with God?*
2. *How are you able to recognize your giants?*
3. *What strategies did you use to defeat your giants?*
4. *How have you allowed your giants to interfere with your adventure?*

CHAPTER 6

Faith and Trust

Faith is believing that God can do it
Trust is believing that God will do it

When you embark on an adventure with God, you have to pack plenty of faith. Hebrews 11:1 states that faith is the substance of things hoped for, the evidence of things not seen. It is the expectation God is going to do everything he said he would. God knows your needs and doesn't want you to focus on your situation. Faith is what you will have to embrace despite the disappointments you may experience.

I have always considered myself to have strong faith in God. I had what people in the church call, "crazy" faith. It's the faith can withstand any trial or tribulation. Surely this faith was going to deliver me from my predicament. Everything was going to be ok because this was not the first instance of something unexpectedly occurring in my life. So, with my "crazy" faith, I prayed to God everything was going to work out for the best. Faith dictated my situation would soon turn around.

My faith was being tested, and I was failing! As time passed and I couldn't see anything happening, my faith turned to doubt and began to fade. I began to question God more and more. I was engaged in a "valley" experience and couldn't understand why my situation was still the same. What was different? In my opinion, God was not moving fast enough. Maybe it was because I really didn't understand why this was happening. Or perhaps it was because I felt my prayers were not being answered.

No one wants to wake up in turmoil. We think we are prepared for storms by studying scripture. But when the crisis actually appears, our faith may start to fizzle. This makes me think of Jesus walking on the sea. When his disciples saw this, they thought it was a ghost and became fearful. Peter said, *"Lord, if it's you, command me to come to you on the water."* "*Come*," Jesus said. Peter got down out of the boat, walked on the water and went toward Jesus. *"But when he saw the wind, he was afraid, and beginning to sink he cried out, "Lord, save me."* Jesus immediately reached out his hand and took hold of him, saying, *"O you of little faith, why did you doubt?"* (Matthew 14:22-31). This verse gives a glimpse into the faith Jesus wants us to have.

Peter and I have a lot in common. Although I was not sinking in "water", I found myself sinking in depression, self pity, fear, grief and hopelessness. My adventure started by me taking Jesus' hand, relishing the fact everything was going to work out. However, I took my eyes off Jesus, focusing on my circumstances, and became afraid. Many of us may have the same experience. Your situations cause you to lose focus. Your faith weakens and fear enters your spirit. It's a bad report from the doctor. It's your child on the streets. It's the months that have passed and you still don't have a job. It's the bills piling up. It's the certified letter that your home is going into foreclosure. The list is endless. Powerless, you begin to sink. What I admire about Peter is he had the sense to realize:

- He was sinking
- He needed Jesus

What a prime example of what needs to be done on an adventure with God. Recognize those external factors which may cause you to sink. Depression can overpower you. Stress will infiltrate your body, causing you to be submerged. Worry can weigh you down like an anchor and quickly send you to the sea of hopelessness. As soon as you recognize the signs, a distress call has to be made. When Peter called out, immediately Jesus stretched forth his hand and grabbed him. Jesus then asked Peter, *"Why did you doubt?"* That's what so amazing about embarking on an adventure with God. Jesus is there to stretch forth his hand in your hour of need. Faith dictates there is no room for doubt.

Trust

When God chooses you to embark on an adventure with Him, He wants you to trust He has your best interests at heart. Faith must be supported with trust. Faith is a noun. It is something you have. Trust is a verb, it is something you have to DO. I knew I had to trust God to bring me out of my situation, but it was hard for me to trust the way He was doing it!

I was talking to my daughter one evening and she asked me if I really trust God, because she did not see it exhibited in my walk. She saw in me a person giving up and not believing God for a breakthrough. Like many, I trust God for some things and doubt Him for others. I wish there was an explanation for this. I knew God was taking me on an adventure where I had to fully put my trust in Him. I was just having a problem with *how* He was taking me on it. Faith must be supported with trust. Trust is something you must do, but I wasn't "doing" it. Doubt started to overtake my trust and I found myself trusting in things not ordained by God. For example, I have always said, "God is a God of promotion and not demotion." During my adventure, I kept repeating these words. I believed with all my heart God was going to restore me to the position I previously held. When it didn't happen immediately, I found myself starting to negotiate with God. My original "trust" was put on the backburner and I began to ask God for any position, even if it meant a demotion. My actions were proof of dwindling trust. I was willing to settle for something not part of God's plan. Since I was not demonstrating trust in my daily walk, I needed to re-evaluate my position with God and take "me" out of the equation.

In 1 Samuel 8 the Israelites wanted a king so they would be like everyone else. Although the request displeased Samuel, he still took it to God. God told Samuel to do everything they said, for in reality, it was Him (God) who they were rejecting. That was me. I wanted my situation to change so I could be like everyone else. I wanted to be validated by returning to my old way of life. Everything was familiar and comfortable. God wanted me to go on this adventure with Him with no distractions, but that wasn't enough for me. I finally realized God has to set his children apart. We are unique. God has an ultimate plan for our lives, a plan that is going to force us to fully put our faith and trust in Him.

Reflection Question

1. *Think about the situation you are currently in. How does faith and trust play a role on your adventure?*
2. *Where is your focus on your adventure? Is it lined up with the will of God? Is your focus interfering with your faith and/or trust?*
3. *How do you react when you don't have evidence of God "moving" on your behalf?*
4. *On a scale of 1 – 10, where would you rate your faith at this moment? Your trust? What can you do to increase it?*

CHAPTER 7

The Pits

Pit – A covered or concealed excavation in the ground, serving as a trap.

I remember vividly the beginning of my adventure. I felt someone had thrown me in a pit and completely forgot about me. I felt so alone and could not understand why a person I trusted would do this to me. I became bitter, wanting to get even with everyone who had known about my predicament and didn't warn me. I wanted revenge on my "so called" friends who turned their back on me in my hour of need. I was not in a good place and felt the need to lash out at anything or anyone who came in contact with me.

In Genesis 37, Joseph's father has presented him with a coat of many colors to indicate his love for his son and the fact he was born after Jacob was very old. Joseph was not perfect, but God chose him to embark on an adventure with Him whose purpose would not be known until the end of Genesis 50.

One day Joseph goes to the fields to tell his brothers about his dream that one day, they would bow down to him. This made Joseph's brothers, who already held hostility toward him, hate him even more. Be aware of the fact that when God places something in your heart - a dream, an aspiration, a specific purpose - you cannot share it with everyone. When you embark on your adventure with God, you are going to have those "haters" in your life who want to know why God chose **you** to embark on your adventure. If you tell them the dreams God is placing in your heart, they will become angry and what to find a way abolish the dream and the dreamer. I knew there were seeds God had planted in my spirit I couldn't share with anyone else. I knew there were going to be naysayers. There were going to be those to tell me, "You're crazy! Your dreams don't make sense. There is no way anything good is going to happen for you!" If I was going to make my dreams come true and be obedient to the calling God had placed on my life, I would have to remain silent.

Joseph's brothers become jealous of him and decide they are going to throw him in a pit. (Genesis 37:24). Then, they surmised, let's see what will become of his dreams. I now know it was part of God's divine purpose I was thrown into my pit. Although it was cold and desolate, I knew it was a temporary pit God was going to deliver me from. This was my "valley" experience, the beginning of my evolution. It was a place where God could get my attention and speak in a still, small voice I could understand. No, it was not comfortable, but it was necessary. I realized everything God had planted in my spirit was about to come to pass. Dreams were going to become a reality. Assignments were going to be completed. My pit became my "period of preparation." I began keeping a journal of goals and created a checklist. I focused on the dreams that had become deferred in my life. I listed areas in my life I knew I needed to work on. Everything was now beginning to make more sense.

Joseph is taken to Egypt and sold to Potiphar who recognized the favor of God upon him (Genesis 39:1-6). The benefits that come with favor include an improved relationship with God, unwavering faith, needs being met according to God's promises and undeserved grace and mercy. When you have found favor with God, there are going to be people who will want to kill you spiritually because they don't want to see you advancing in the kingdom of God. Hold your head up despite your situation. People will recognize the favor of God is also upon you and that you will not allow your situation to dictate a negative disposition.

Potiphar's wife wanted to engage in a sexual relationship with Joseph (Genesis 39:7-20). In the midst of your adventure, you cannot allow the enemy to entice you to do something contrary to God's will. Remember, the enemy comes to kill, steal and destroy. It is so easy to sin and fall short of God's word. You will rationalize, "I'm in this crisis, and I might as well make the most of it!" No, renew the moral fiber in you that tells you to resist the enemy and his tricks. Joseph stood his ground and told her he would not sin against God by doing such a terrible thing. That has to be your stance – no matter how attractive the circumstance, I will not sin against God.

Joseph is accused of rape and thrown into jail. Even in jail, God helped Joseph and was good to him (Genesis 39:21-23). That's what so awesome about our adventure. In the midst of our storm, we will still experience the goodness of God. God allows the jailer to find favor with Joseph, who in turn makes him the head jailer! There's that word again – favor! It never leaves you, surrounding you wherever your situation leads you. The jailer did not worry about anything because it was evident the Lord was with Joseph and made him successful in all he did.

While in jail, Joseph meets a baker and a butler, who both have dreams (Genesis 40). God has given Joseph the ability to interpret their dreams. Joseph interprets the baker's dream and lets him know in 3 days he will die. He informs the butler that in three days the king would pardon him and he will become his personal servant. All Joseph requested from the butler was when these good things happen, he remembers him. I know how Joseph felt when the butler is released from jail and forgets about him. There were people who I felt were in a position to help me who totally forgot about me. I placed my faith in people instead of placing it where it should have been – in God.

Two years later, the king of Egypt had a dream no one was able to interpret. It was then the butler remembered Joseph and mentioned to the king there was a Hebrew who was able to interpret dreams (Genesis 41). Joseph informs the king he cannot interpret dreams by his own might, but only by the power of God. Notice that once Joseph is brought out of jail, albeit 2 years later, he is still about the Master's business. He is not bitter about the butler not keeping his word. He is not angry he was thrown in jail for something he didn't do. He acknowledges the power of God. I had to remind myself about God's absolute authority. Nothing could happen in my life that He did not allow. It finally dawned on me that everything I was going through had been pre-approved by God. Be patient. It may be days, weeks, months or even years. God has not forgotten about you.

Joseph interprets the king's dream and is made governor over all Egypt (Genesis 41:41). Talk about promotion. This is what God is doing for you while you are on your adventure. He is elevating you. Follow God's plan, embrace your situation, and maintain your character.

Events happened just as Joseph interpreted. There was a famine in Egypt and it is at this time Joseph's brothers enter the picture again (Genesis 42-45). They had to go to Joseph who eventually reveals his identity to them. Little did they know that the one they threw in a pit was the one who was going to be a blessing to them.

After all that Joseph had been through on his adventure, he chose to help his brothers. He did not hold anything against them or throw it in their face that, indeed, they bowed down to him. When your adversaries see you elevated, they may assume you are going to pay them back for what they did. Realize that, like Joseph, you are in a better place because of what God allowed them to do. Joseph lets his brothers know that although they may have meant everything they had done to him for evil, God had turned it around for good (Genesis 50:19). The good was not just for Joseph, but also for the number of people who were blessed as a result of Joseph's adventure. Through your trials, not only are you being blessed, but others can be blessed also. How awesome is that?

Reflection Questions

1. *Reflect on your life and where you are right now. Are you happy? Do you feel you are where you're supposed to be spiritually? Are there dreams you have given up on because they seem out of reach? Why?*
2. *What was the reaction from others when you shared your dreams with them? How did this affect you emotionally and spiritually?*
3. *What are some of the "pits" you have been in or are currently in? How do you view them?*
4. *How do you view the people who have set traps for you?*
5. *How will you handle the people who come back to you? Will you forgive and forget? Will you be a blessing to them? Will you hold a grudge?*

CHAPTER 8

Patience is a Virtue

Patience - the capacity to accept or tolerate delay, trouble, or suffering without getting angry or upset.

The demand for instant gratification is soaking into every aspect of our lives. We use instant cereal, can obtain loans instantly on line, and can buy "fast passes" to jump to the front of a line. The list is endless. We get upset with technology when it doesn't move fast enough or a red light if it is prolonged. We grow impatient if we have to wait too long at a restaurant. Yes, we all lack patience. The faster the better!

I remember at the beginning of my adventure how I kept wondering how much longer I would have to endure my pain. Deep down, I knew God had a blessing for me. I just didn't want to wait for it. In my mind, God was not moving fast enough. I wanted my ordeal to be over instantly. I didn't feel I had the strength I needed to continue on an adventure and was ready to take a bullet train to my destination.

When you set out on an adventure with God, it is not about your timetable, but God's. God told Abram (Abraham) he would have a son and his descendants would outnumber the stars. (Genesis 15) Abram believed the Lord who was pleased with him. The problem became "time" which becomes your enemy. As it slowly ticked away, Sarah is advancing in age so they decided to jump ahead of God. You may feel the need to assist God when He is not moving according to your timetable. It had already been ten years for Abraham and Sarah and she realized her biological clock is winding down. In their mind, time is of the essence. It's been a week, a month, a year, and you still don't see God moving. That's when you decide to help him out. Sarah allows her husband to sleep with her Egyptian slave and reasoned that if she has a child, it will be theirs. From that union a son was born. But what did God say? The child that God was going to bless them with was to be born from Sarah.

Before you think negatively about Abraham and Sarah, examine the facts. Abraham was advancing in age. His wife Sara was the already past childbearing years. The first thing Abraham does is question God. Isn't that your first response, especially when the facts don't add up? God tells you something miraculous is going to happen in your life, and you begin to wonder how God is going to do it. The fact God planted the seed in your heart is never enough. Your doubts become your obstacles. How is this going to happen? I'm advancing in age. I don't have the required education. My background is lousy. I've always been told I would never amount to anything. You have to get pass these excuses and realize if God said it, it will happen. Time is never an issue with God and shouldn't be with you.

Abram (Abraham) was ninety-nine years old when the Lord appeared to him again and reminded him He would give him more descendant than could be counted. God changes his name to Abraham and informs him his descendants will become great nations. How was God going to keep His promise against these odds? Again, Abraham decides to help God and suggests Ishmael, his child with the Egyptian slave, inherit the promise. Essentially, Abraham was giving away his future heirs' blessings. When you become impatient and try to reason with God, you may never know the blessing you and your future generations will miss out on. God again informs Abraham he and Sarah will have a son, his name will be Isaac, and an everlasting promise would be made to him and his descendants.

God could have given Abraham a son instantly. God could give you everything you ask Him for instantly, but what purpose would that serve. You would become spoiled and always expect instant gratification. God wants to build your resilience up. Your patience is building up your faith, your trust and your dependence on Him. You cannot allow your waiting period to make you become hopeless, discouraged, and want to throw in the towel. Believe me, God will come through. Eventually, Abraham and Sarah have a son, just as God had promised.

The key to embarking on an adventure with God is to realize your patience is vital. A lack of patience may cause you to miss out on the things God wants you to experience. Wait expectantly. This means you can't give up or stop believing. You may feel time is not on your side, but in reality, it is. *Wait patiently for the LORD. Be brave and courageous. Yes, wait patiently for the LORD (Psalm 27:14).*

Reflection Questions

1. *How has your patience been tested?*
2. *Like Abraham, have you ever tried to "help" God out? What were the results?*
3. *Have you been waiting on the Lord in a particular area of your life? What is it that keeps you from giving up?*
4. *Are there excuses preventing you from waiting on God to move? How can you delete them?*

CHAPTER 9

The Holy Spirit Packs a Powerful Punch

Holy Spirit – The spirit and presence of God as part of a person's religious experience.

A boxer has the ability to size up his opponent and deliver a powerful punch that overtakes his challenger. Like a fighter's mighty blow, the Holy Spirit's "punch" is crucial. It has the ability to stop your adversaries from attacking you in your most vulnerable areas. The Holy Spirit has many roles which will build up your endurance while on your adventure with God. Without it, you would experience a spiritual knock out.

The Holy Spirit has the ability to guide you, leading you on a path free from obstacles and challenges that would otherwise make travel impossible. While the Israelites were on their adventure, God went ahead of them in a pillar of cloud to guide them on their way by day and a pillar of fire by night (Exodus 13:21). They became dependent on these pillars – cloud and fire. They knew that as long as they were there, God was with them, directing their path. When the cloud or fire was not evident, they would set up camp until it reappeared. On our adventure, we don't have a cloud or fire leading us, but God left something even better, the Holy Spirit. It is impossible to follow God without being led by His spirit.

The Holy Spirit is the power of God working within you. It renews your strength when you are ready to throw in the towel. This is when your endurance kicks in. When Jesus appeared to His disciples the final time after His resurrection, He told them to stay in the city until the Holy Spirit came and filled them with power from heaven (Luke 24:49). He didn't want them speaking from "self" but from the spirit.

He wanted them to be powerful in their daily walk and talk, which is what the Holy Spirit does. During your adventure you will have to be an example to someone else who may be experiencing hardships in their life. Embarking on an adventure with God means the gifts you receive will make you courageous, bold, confident and insightful. As you move toward a greater relationship with God, use these gifts to spread His message and work toward your dreams and aspirations.

The Holy Spirit becomes your counselor and teacher on your adventure. There are so many things you are going to become knowledgeable of. God does not want you to be ignorant. Your awareness comes from studying the word of God and allowing him to increase your understanding regarding His purpose for your life. You need God's timing and power to be truly informed on your adventure. There are some questions that may never be answered:

- Why is this happening to me?
- What did I do to deserve this?
- How will I ever get over this mountain?
- Where is God leading me?
- When is this going to be over?

The good news is, eventually all your question will become periods.

Satan's plan of attack on the Christian is to cause a separation between man and God through sin; therefore, the Holy Spirit will convict you of right and wrong. It will not allow you to do anything in direct conflict with God or His word. God also does not want you to be ignorant of the tricks of Satan. *"Lest Satan should get an advantage of us; for we are not ignorant of his devices."* (2 Corinthians 2:12). Satan has an infinite amount of tricks and traps he uses to quench the Holy Spirit. I recall his voice speaking to me quietly to impair my spiritual life by planting seeds of doubt, disgust and discouragement. I was offered a job (after a year of looking) that was going to interfere with the assignment God had for me. Satan knew I wanted a job so he presented me with the perfect position. I prayed and asked God to allow his spirit to lead me in making my final decision. The spirit revealed to me that God was preparing to promote me in my personal life and ministry. Satan was going to do anything to stop this promotion. Since I allowed the Holy Spirit to dwell in me, I knew I had to turn down the offer. As a saint of God, I knew the importance of continually asking the Holy

Spirit to lead, guide, and assist me in my decisions. Satan is going to paint a picture for you that will be so lucrative, it will be hard to resist it. Although your eyes and mind may be clouded, it becomes important to pray and seek the truth before making any final decisions.

<u>Reflection Questions</u>

1. *What has the Holy Spirit revealed to you during your adventure?*
2. *Is there another spirit you are fighting with that is in direct conflict with God's Spirit?*
   How are you counteracting this spirit?
3. *What knowledge have you gained as a result of your adventure?*
4. *Where is the Holy Spirit leading you? Is this the path you thought you were going to embark on?*
5. *Are you fully following the will of God or your own will? Why/ Why not?*

CHAPTER 10

Integrity Counts!

Integrity - the quality of being honest and having strong moral principles; moral uprightness

Are you a person of integrity? Do your actions display truth as a testimony of faith in your daily walk? As you surround yourself with others, do you tend to take on the characteristics of those people? There are so many temptations you will face when you try to lead a life of integrity. God expects us to exhibit integrity, which means it is the measurement of our character. As Christians, we can't conform to our environment. We can't become the type of person that changes their direction every time the wind blows. There comes a time when we have to be bold through our words and deeds. Everything we do as a child of God must be done in integrity, frankness, and candor, as we are representing the most High God! When we say we follow God and His Word, do our actions show we do? There is no better example of this than in the book of Daniel.

The book of Daniel recalls the story of how Daniel and his friends are taken captive from their homes in Judah and living in exile. Part of Daniel's captivity included the expectation he take on the characteristics and culture of the people he was now associated with. Daniel had strong faith and lived his life according to the will of God. As a captive, Daniel's first test of integrity was his refusal to eat the royal food offered to him. For many, that probably would not be a big deal. When you think about it, it's only food. But, Daniel had integrity. According to Jewish law, it was not permissible to eat certain foods, and Daniel was determined not to defile himself. While on your adventure, you are going to be offered things in opposition with what God has already pre-ordained. This is when your integrity really counts. You have to have strong moral principles and refuse to participate in anything in indirect conflict with God.

Daniel 6 introduces King Darius and the favor Daniel has found with him. Daniel is elevated, but his elevation brings jealousy from the administrators and high officers in King Darius' court. Daniel 6:4 states the other men tried to find something wrong with the way Daniel did his work for the king, but they could not accuse him of anything wrong. Daniel was honest, faithful, and full of integrity. The only thing they could think of to trap him with was the fact he was a prayer warrior. They realized they would never be able to bring any charges against Daniel, unless it had to do with his faith. The governors go to King Darius to convince him to set up a decree that for 30 days no one be allowed to pray to any god except him. The irony of this is that while on your adventure, the enemy will use people to stop your advancement in the kingdom unbeknownst even to them.

Daniel obviously was not concerned about the law. He heard about it, but he didn't stress or try to figure out how to pray secretly so he wouldn't get caught. No, he went upstairs in the window that faced Jerusalem, bowed down, and prayed to God. What boldness Daniel showed. This is a prime example of the boldness to possess. You do not have to compromise your integrity because the enemy thinks he has trapped you and there are no other choices. Keep doing what is right and acceptable in the sight of God. If Daniel had not gone and prayed, as was his custom, he would have allowed his enemies to "win" and could have missed out on the blessings God had in store for him. If you allow your enemies to succeed, you may miss out on your blessings.

I realized on my adventure that despite my circumstances, I had to stand firm in my belief God was going to deliver me. Yes, I was going through a difficult time, but I knew I had to realize it was only a temporary situation. I maintained my integrity by consistently serving God. I demonstrated my faithfulness by trusting and obeying the calling on my life. I embraced my Christian values so they would be exhibited to everyone I came in contact with. I knew I had to practice what I preached, which is really what integrity is all about.

Daniel is thrown into a pit of lions to be executed. Here is another example of Daniel's integrity in the face of death. He put his trust in

God knowing he was in the hands of God. Like Daniel, realize that God will deliver you in unimaginable ways. It would be premature to give up to the pressures of others. God shut the lion's mouth for Daniel and He will do the same for you. This is what is so awesome about our faithfulness to God during our adventure and our refusal to compromise our integrity. He will rescue you from your "pit". It was Daniel's faith in God and his integrity that kept him from being harmed. It is these same principles that will deliver you.

Reflection Questions

1. *What do you believe people are thinking about when they observe your behavior while on your adventure? How are you maintaining your integrity?*
2. *What Godly "trap" could someone set for you?*
3. *Have you ever been thrown in a 'pit'? How did God rescue you?*

CHAPTER 11

Stand Your Ground - Refuse to Compromise

Compromise: a change that can make something worse when it is not done for a good reason.

Compromise is crucial in any relationship: family, friends, co-workers and the like. In these types of examples, it is important to know which battles to fight and those worth conceding to. I remember arguing with my husband over what color we should paint the walls in our bedroom. Deep down, I did like the color he chose, but I didn't want to give in. I finally realized it was ok to listen to what he was trying to say and concede. My ability to compromise in this situation led to a happy ending. But there are times when compromise is not an alternative. This is most notable when it comes to the Word of God. There are certain truths the bible teaches that are not even up for debate. When you begin to compromise the truth and bend on honorable beliefs, it can become spiritually lethal. Satan will present you with eye appealing decoys to take you off your adventure. By the time you delve in the decoy, at some point you realize the trick of the enemy got you off track.

During my adventure I found myself ready to compromise. I was ready to ignore the word implanted in my spirit, just so my storm would be over. Maybe this was how my adventure was supposed to end. Forget about faith the size of a mustard seed. I didn't see it working for me. Forget about praying fervently. I would just pray when I wanted to. Forget about focusing on the promises of God. I didn't see any of them being kept on my behalf. I would just let Satan win this round! I would settle for any position even if it was not ordained by God. Yes, I could compromise – I was ready to compromise.

In Daniel 3, King Nebuchadnezzar has set up a golden image he wants everyone to bow down to. Refusal to do so meant being thrown into a fiery furnace. The enemy wants us to "bow down" to "golden images'. These images are the things the world offers contrary to God's will. Word came to the king that three Hebrew boys, Shadrach, Meshach, and Abednego, refused to bow. On our adventure with God, there are going to be situations when we face fiery furnaces. There will be furnaces of criticism, furnaces of intimidation, furnaces of hatred, furnaces of stress, and furnaces of trials. It is normal to want to bypass these furnaces, but that won't always be the case.

King Nebuchadnezzar hears that Shadrach, Meshach and Abednego refuse to bow down to the golden image and falls into a rage. They are brought before him and informed he is willing to give them another chance. He reminds them that their refusal will result in immediately being thrown into the fiery furnace and asks what god would be able to rescue them from his power? But the three Hebrew boys stood firm, refusing to compromise. They could have easily reasoned the following:

- I'll bow down this one time and ask God for forgiveness.
- It will be ok. The Word does tell us to obey those who have rule over us.
- We will just be like everyone around us and bow down. God knows our hearts.
- If something happens to us, how is God going to continue to use us?

It's so easy to make excuses and try to justify them. The three Hebrew Boys didn't make excuses, give the king an apology, or try to reason with him. No, they took a stand! Taking a stand, even when others don't agree with it, prevents them from controlling you. You don't want your testimony erased. How can you minister to family, friends, and/or strangers of the power of God if you have not experienced it? Your position not to compromise is saying to God, "I trust you and believe what your Word says. I will stand firm, despite the furnaces I face."

Shadrach, Meshach, and Abednego informed the king they did not need to defend themselves before him. They did not need to have a caucus, a discussion, a gab fest, or take a vote on the matter. NO. *"If we are thrown into the blazing furnace, the God whom we serve is able to rescue us from your power."* (Daniel 3:17). This statement demonstrates their firm position. We should be faithful to serve God whether He intervenes on our behalf or not. They inform Nebuchadnezzar they would not bow down. It is this same power that we must use when faced with the possibility of being thrown into a fiery furnace. On your adventure, refuse to compromise, even when you don't know the outcome.

Nebuchadnezzar became furious and commands the furnace be heated seven times hotter than usual. He orders some of the strongest men of his army to bind the Hebrew boys. Is that what your furnace feels like? Not only are you in the furnace, but you are also bound! Bound by your situations; be it physical, mental or spiritual. The key is to focus on the one who is able to set you to be free.

Nebuchadnezzar jumps up in amazement at the sight of seeing four men walking around in the fire, unbound and unharmed. Even though the ropes that had them bound burned off, the fire didn't touch them (Daniel 3:25). Not a hair on their heads was singed and their clothing was not scorched. They did not even smell of smoke. When God delivers you from your fiery furnace, the enemy will be amazed you are not carrying around the evidence of your ordeal. They will realize, just as Nebuchadnezzar did, that God's power was available to rescue them. If you compromise, just to bypass your fiery furnace, you will not have the tools needed to face other furnaces you will surely encounter. Deliverance from your fiery furnace will give confirmation to others that there are no other gods like God. He protected, comforted, and ultimately rewarded them through promotion. Face your fiery furnace and stand firm. Your destiny is not in the hands of others, but in God's.

Reflection Questions

1. *Have you felt the need to compromise while on your adventure? What was the source of your need to compromise?*
2. *There are many valid reasons the Hebrew Boys could have bowed down to the golden image. What reasons would cause you to "bow down"?*
3. *What fiery furnaces have you or are you being confronted with?*

4. *The three Hebrew Boys stood firm in their decision not to bow down. How firm are you when you take a stand for the Lord?*
5. *Give examples of how God delivered you from your fiery furnaces and how others were blessed as a result.*

CHAPTER 12

God's Promises Are Still In Effect

Promise – A statement telling someone that you will definitely do something or that something will definitely happen in the future.

There are literally thousands of promises in the bible God wants you to build your spiritual foundation on. Some promises may speak to your spirit more than others. The amazing thing is you can always count on God's promises. In the beginning of my adventure, I was more focused on my situation and really cared less about God's promises. I was not in a good place spiritually or mentally. How were God's promises going to get me a job? How were God's promises going to pay my bills? How were God's promises going to open the many doors being shut in my face daily? Basically, how were God's promises going to change my situation? God's promises were the last thing on my mind.

I remember walking one morning and engaging in a conversation with God. I was angry and felt it was the perfect moment for me to pour my feelings out before Him. God revealed to me that He had a plan for my life. There was still one tiny problem – I was not part of the planning process! How can anyone make plans for me without my consent? I recalled the scripture states, *"For I know the plans I have for you, declares the LORD, plans to prosper you and not to harm you, plans to give you hope and a future."* (Jeremiah 29:11) This made me realize that, although I was not part of the planning process, the plans God had for me were not going to destroy me, but enhance me. This was a promise!

I finally learned to revamp my thinking. I could not embark on an adventure and not focus on God's promises. The road will not be easy, but it will be within your capabilities and limits. He will not put anything on you that you cannot bear. God promises that He will direct your path if you:

- Trust him – Lord I don't know what you are doing in my life right now. I am confused, not fully understanding why I am on this adventure right now, but I do trust that you know what is best for me.
- Lean not unto you own understanding – Lord, I know that I don't fully understand the thoughts you have for me. My understanding is finite but you are infinite; therefore, I am putting myself secondary to you.
- Acknowledge Him – Lord, I acknowledge you as the Supreme Being. You are the Lord that created heaven and earth and I acknowledge you as the one true and living God.

During your adventure, there will be days you become weak and want to give up. You will question yourself, "Is this is really for me?" Trust me, your strength will waste away and you will want to give up. It is at those times God's promises come into full effect. Think about a marathon. A marathon runner does not just wake up on the day of the race and start running. It takes preparation. God has prepared you for your adventure. Only He can give you the endurance to complete it.

I have listed a few promises to help you while you are on your adventure with God:

- ***But my God shall supply all your need according to his riches in glory by Christ Jesus (Philippians 4:19.)***
- ***When thou passest through the waters, I will be with thee; and through the rivers, they shall not overflow thee: when thou walkest through the fire, thou shalt not be burned; neither shall the flame kindle upon thee (Isaiah 43:2***).
- ***Trust in the LORD with all thine heart; and lean not unto thine own understanding. In all thy ways acknowledge him, and he shall direct thy paths. (Proverbs 3:5-6).***
- ***But they that wait upon the LORD shall renew their strength; they shall mount up with wings as eagles; they shall run, and not be weary; and they shall walk, and not faint (Isaiah 40:31).***

- ***"I am leaving you with a gift—peace of mind and heart. And the peace I give is a gift the world cannot give. So don't be troubled or afraid (John 14:27).***
- ***God won't let me be tried or tempted beyond what I can endure (1 Corinthians 10:13).***
- ***For the Lord my God will be with me, wherever I go (Joshua 1:9).***
- ***God will keep me in perfect peace if my mind is 'stayed' on Him (Isaiah 26:3).***
- ***God has created good works for me to walk in, today (Ephesians 2:10).***

On your adventure remind yourself daily about God's promises. Allow them to penetrate your mind, heart and soul. It is these promises that will sustain throughout your adventure.

Reflection Questions

1. *What are some of the promises of God you have found yourself focusing on?*
2. *Are you allowing the promises of God to guide you on your adventure? Why/Why not?*
3. *Meditate on the three of the listed promises of God in this chapter. What is God trying to instill in you through these promises?*

FINAL THOUGHTS

I could never imagine my life now if I had not allowed God to take me out of my comfort zone and into an adventure with Him. I have learned so much about myself and have grown spiritually as a result. I know there is nothing too hard for God because I have seen miraculous events happen in my life. At my lowest point, I felt His presence, ensuring me everything was going to work out for my good. I learned to surrender totally to God, and as a result, our relationship has grown to unimaginable heights.

That's what the results of an adventure with God should be. *And we know that in all things God works for the good of those who love him, and who been called according to his purpose. (Romans 8:28).* It is so reassuring to know everything you have been through or going through is essentially an adventure you have been called to embark on. Everything is going to work out for your good. You may not see it at the time, but it will come full circle.

If I was to offer any advice to make your adventure easier, it would be the following:

- Take time to notice the "little" things that you have taken for granted.
- Don't take yourself too seriously. Take a "chill pill".
- Volunteer. It will make you realize how blessed you really are.
- Never become too comfortable where you are.
- Strike up a conversation with a complete stranger.
- Choose:
    - Choose to be happy.
    - Choose to make the most of your adventure.
    - Choose to laugh at loud.

    - Choose to wake up every morning with a purpose.
- Keep a journal. When you reflect on it, you will be amazed at how much you have grown spiritually, emotionally and physically.
- Surround yourself with men and women with Godly character. You will find your adventure much more enjoyable.

Moses never wanted to lead the Israelites out of bondage. Noah did not set out to build an ark. David never dreamed of being King. The 12 disciples didn't fully realize who they were following when they were first chosen. Job never knew why he lost everything, only to receive double for his trouble. Joshua could have never imagined he would lead the children of Israel to the Promised Land. What do all these people have in common? They were chosen to embark on their adventure because God had a plan for their life, just like He has for yours. You are part of an elite club and being transformed for a destiny that no one can fulfill but you. Now you know why you were chosen to *Embark on an Adventure with God*. Your steps have been ordered toward the spiritual fulfillment that will forever enhance your life. May God continue to bless and keep you is my prayer.

ACKNOWLEDGEMENTS

I want to first thank God for uprooting me from the familiar and using me for a purpose that far exceeded anything that I could have ever imagined. I was led down a path that was unfamiliar, but necessary for the fulfillment of the plans you had for my life.

Thank you to my wonderful parents, Fred and Fraulyn Baisey, who have supported me in all my endeavors. You taught me to love the Lord with all my heart and to acknowledge Him in everything I do. You trained me up, "in the way that I should go" and I have never departed from it. I hope that I have made you proud.

Thank you to my daughters, Kristina and Kathryn Jackson. You are my greatest accomplishment. Never forget how proud I am of you. To my two sisters, Kathleen and Katrice. Thank you for allowing me to be myself and never allowing me to have a pity party. I love you guys so much.

A special thank you to my Inter-grated Missionary Church Family. I have always felt your continued prayers and unconditional love and support. Montre, thank you for obeying God's word and speaking life into an idea that has blossomed into this project.

Richie, Fred, Vance Sr. & II, Wayne Sr. & II, Tiffany, and Glenn III & IV– you guys rock! A huge shout out to all my family and friends who encouraged me during a difficult period in my life. Your positive words will forever be hidden in my heart.

Alesia, thank you for helping me get this project completed. You never allowed me to become complacent.

To my wonderful husband, Marvin Jackson. As a little girl, I knew that one day we would become one. I didn't realize at the time what God was implanting in my life. I considered it to be a childhood crush, but it was so much more. It was the beginning of a union that would become the fulfillment of God's plans for our life. You have truly been my rock and exemplify what it means to be a strong man. Your strength is the glue that holds our family together. Thank you so much for loving me unconditionally. I love you.

Printed in the United States
By Bookmasters